PUBLIC HEALTH IN THE 21ST CENTURY

NATIONAL STRATEGY AND ACTION PLAN FOR COMBATING ANTIBIOTIC RESISTANT BACTERIA

Public Health in the 21st Century

Additional books in this series can be found on Nova's website under the Series tab.

Additional e-books in this series can be found on Nova's website under the e-book tab.

PUBLIC HEALTH IN THE 21ST CENTURY

NATIONAL STRATEGY AND ACTION PLAN FOR COMBATING ANTIBIOTIC RESISTANT BACTERIA

ANTHONY PHILLIPS
EDITOR

nova publishers
New York

Library of Congress Cataloging-in-Publication Data

ISBN: 978-1-63483-072-0

Published by Nova Science Publishers, Inc. † New York

CONTENTS

PREFACE

The discovery of antibiotics in the early 20th century fundamentally transformed human and veterinary medicine. Antibiotics now save millions of lives each year in the United States and around the world. The rise of antibiotic-resistant bacterial strains, however, represents a serious threat to public health and the economy. If the effectiveness of antibiotics (drugs that kill or inhibit the growth of bacteria) is lost, we will no longer be able to reliably and rapidly treat bacterial infections, including bacterial pneumonias, foodborne illnesses, and healthcare-associated infections. As more strains of bacteria become resistant to an ever-larger number of antibiotics, our drug choices have become increasingly limited and more expensive and, in some cases, nonexistent. In a world with few effective antibiotics, modern medical advances such as surgery, transplants, and chemotherapy may no longer be viable due to the threat of infection. This book presents the national strategy and action plan for combating antibiotic-resistant bacteria.

In: National Strategy
Editor: Anthony Phillips

ISBN: 978-1-63483-072-0

Chapter 1

NATIONAL STRATEGY FOR COMBATING ANTIBIOTIC-RESISTANT BACTERIA*

President's Council of Advisors on Science and Technology

Vision: The United States will work domestically and internationally to prevent, detect, and control illness and death related to infections caused by antibiotic- resistant bacteria by implementing measures to mitigate the emergence and spread of antibiotic resistance and ensuring the continued availability of therapeutics for the treatment of bacterial infections.

EXECUTIVE SUMMARY

The discovery of antibiotics in the early 20th century fundamentally transformed human and veterinary medicine. Antibiotics now save millions of lives each year in the United States and around the world. The rise of antibiotic-resistant bacterial strains, however, represents a serious threat to public health and the economy. The Centers for Disease Control and Prevention (CDC) estimates that annually, at least two million illnesses and 23,000 deaths are caused by antibiotic-resistant bacteria in the United States

* This is an edited, reformatted and augmented version of a document issued by the Executive Office of the President, September 2014.

alone.[1] If the effectiveness of antibiotics (drugs that kill or inhibit the growth of bacteria) is lost, we will no longer be able to reliably and rapidly treat bacterial infections, including bacterial pneumonias, foodborne illnesses, and healthcare-associated infections. As more strains of bacteria become resistant to an ever-larger number of antibiotics, our drug choices have become increasingly limited and more expensive and, in some cases, nonexistent. In a world with few effective antibiotics, modern medical advances such as surgery, transplants, and chemotherapy may no longer be viable due to the threat of infection.

The *National Strategy for Combating Antibiotic Resistant Bacteria* identifies priorities and coordinates investments: to prevent, detect, and control outbreaks of resistant pathogens recognized by CDC as urgent or serious threats, including carbapenem-resistant *Enterobacteriaceae* (CRE), methicillin-resistant *Staphylococcus aureus* (MRSA), ceftriaxoneresistant *Neisseria gonorrhoeae*, and *Clostridium difficile,* which is naturally resistant to many drugs used to treat other infections and proliferates following administration of antibiotics (Table 1); to ensure continued availability of effective therapies for the treatment of bacterial infections; and to detect and control newly resistant bacteria that emerge in humans or animals. This *National Strategy* is the basis of a 2014 Executive Order on Combating Antibiotic Resistance, as well as a forthcoming *National Action Plan* that directs Federal agencies to accelerate our response to this growing threat to the nation's health and security. The *National Action Plan* will be informed by a report approved by the President's Council of Advisors on Science and Technology (PCAST) on July 11, 2014.

The *National Strategy* outlines five interrelated goals for action by the United States Government in collaboration with partners in healthcare, public health, veterinary medicine, agriculture, food safety, and academic, Federal, and industrial research. The goals include:

1. *Slow the Emergence of Resistant Bacteria and Prevent the Spread of Resistant Infections.* Judicious use of antibiotics in healthcare and agricultural settings is essential to slow the emergence of resistance and extend the useful lifetime of effective antibiotics. Antibiotics are a precious resource, and preserving their usefulness will require cooperation and engagement by healthcare providers, healthcare leaders, pharmaceutical companies, veterinarians, the agricultural industry, and patients. Effective dissemination of information to the public is critical. Prevention of resistance also requires rapid detection

and control of outbreaks, along with regional efforts to control transmission across community and healthcare settings.

2. *Strengthen National One-Health Surveillance Efforts to Combat Resistance.* Antibiotic resistance can arise in bacterial pathogens affecting humans, animals, and the environment. Strengthening detection and control of resistance requires the adoption of a "One-Health" approach that promotes integration of public health and veterinary disease, food, and environmental surveillance. Improved detection can be achieved through appropriate data sharing, enhancement, expansion, and coordination of existing surveillance systems, and creation of a regional laboratory network that provides a standardized platform for resistance testing and advanced capacity for genetic characterization of bacteria including whole genome sequencing.
3. *Advance Development and Use of Rapid and Innovative Diagnostic Tests for Identification and Characterization of Resistant Bacteria.* Today, researchers are taking advantage of new technologies to develop rapid "point-of-need" tests that can be used during a healthcare visit to distinguish between viral and bacterial infections and identify bacterial drug susceptibilities—an innovation that could significantly reduce unnecessary antibiotic use. The availability of new rapid diagnostic tests, combined with ongoing use of culture-based assays to identify new resistance mechanisms, will advance the detection and control of resistant bacteria, including the priority pathogens listed in Table 1.
4. *Accelerate Basic and Applied Research and Development for New Antibiotics, Other Therapeutics, and Vaccines.* Antibiotics that lose their effectiveness for treating human disease through antibiotic resistance must be replaced with new drugs. Alternatives to antibiotics are also needed in agriculture and veterinary medicine. The advancement of drug development requires intensified efforts to boost basic scientific research, facilitate clinical trials of new antibiotics, attract greater private investment, and increase the number of antibiotic drug candidates in the drug-development pipeline. We must also promote the development of other tools to combat resistance, including new and next-generation antibiotics, vaccines, additional therapeutics, and diagnostics.
5. *Improve International Collaboration and Capacities for Antibiotic Resistance Prevention, Surveillance, Control, and Antibiotic Research*

and Development. Recognized by G8 Science Ministers in 2013 as "a major health security challenge of the 21st century," antibiotic resistance is a global problem that requires global solutions. The United States will work in concert with the World Health Organization (WHO), the Food and Agriculture Organization of the United Nations (FAO), the World Organization for Animal Health (OIE), ministries of health and agriculture, and other domestic and international stakeholders to strengthen national and international capacities to detect, monitor, analyze, report and characterize antibiotic resistance; provide resources and incentives to spur the development of therapeutics and diagnostics for use in humans and animals; and strengthen regional networks and global partnerships that help prevent and control the emergence and spread of resistance. The United States will support the development of the WHO *Global Action Plan* to address antimicrobial resistance, strengthen cooperation under the European Union-United States Trans-Atlantic Task Force on Antimicrobial Resistance, promote antibiotic resistance as an international health priority, and mobilize resources for global activities through multilateral venues such as the Global Health Security Agenda.

Taken together, implementation of specific objectives provided under each goal (Table 2) will help reduce the incidence of the priority pathogens listed in Table 1. National targets for reducing serious and urgent threats by 2020 are provided in Table 3.

INTRODUCTION

"Every day we don't act to better protect antibiotics will make it harder and more expensive to address drug resistance in the future. Drug resistance can undermine both our ability to fight infectious diseases and much of modern medicine. Patients undergoing chemotherapy for cancer, dialysis for renal failure, and increasingly common treatments for diseases such as arthritis depend on antibiotics so common infectious complications can be treated effectively."

– Dr. Tom Frieden, MD, MPH, Director U.S. Centers for Disease Control and Prevention.

The discovery of antibiotics in the early 20th century fundamentally transformed human and veterinary medicine. Antibiotics now save millions of lives each year in the United States and around the world. The rise of antibiotic-resistant bacterial strains, however, represents a serious threat to public health and the economy. The CDC estimates that annually at least two million illnesses and 23,000 deaths are caused by antibiotic-resistant bacteria in the United States alone.[1]

As more strains of bacteria become resistant to an ever-larger number of antibiotics, our drug choices will become increasingly limited and expensive and, in some cases, nonexistent. If this trend continues unchecked, a wide range of modern medical procedures, from basic dental care to organ transplants, likely would be accompanied by a much greater risk of developing a difficult-to-treat or untreatable antibiotic infection. The safety of many modern medical procedures is dependent on the ability to treat bacterial infections that can arise as posttreatment complications.

Scope of the National Strategy: "Antibiotic resistance" results from mutations or acquisition of new genes in bacteria that reduce or eliminate the effectiveness of antibiotics. "Antimicrobial resistance" is a broader term that encompasses resistance to drugs to treat infections caused by many different types of pathogens, including bacteria, viruses (e.g., influenza and the human immunodeficiency virus (HIV), parasites (e.g., the parasitic protozoan that causes malaria), and fungi (e.g., *Candida spp.*). While all of these pathogens are dangerous to human health, this *Strategy* focuses on resistance in bacteria that presents a serious or urgent threat to public health.

GUIDING PRINCIPLES

Our approach to combating the emergence and spread of antibiotic resistant bacteria takes into consideration goals and objectives (Table 2) including the following:

- Misuse and over-use of antibiotics in healthcare and food production continue to hasten the development of bacterial drug resistance, leading to loss of efficacy of existing antibiotics;

- Detecting and controlling antibiotic resistance requires the adoption of a "One-Health" approach to disease surveillance that recognizes that resistance can arise in humans, animals, and the environment;
- Implementation of evidence-based infection control practices can prevent the spread of resistant pathogens;
- Interventions are necessary to accelerate private sector investment in the development of therapeutics to treat bacterial infections because current private sector interest in antibiotic development is limited;
- There are opportunities to use innovations and new technologies—including whole genome sequencing, metagenomics, and bioinformatic approaches—to develop next-generation tools to strengthen human and animal health, including:
  - Point-of-need diagnostic tests to distinguish rapidly between bacterial and viral infections as well as identify bacterial drug susceptibilities
  - New antibiotics and other therapies that provide much needed treatment options for those infected with resistant bacterial strains;
- Antibiotic resistance is a global health problem that requires international attention and collaboration, because bacteria do not recognize borders.

GOALS AND OBJECTIVES

With these principles in mind, the *Strategy* lays out five interrelated goals that guide collaborative action by the U.S. Government in partnership with foreign governments, individuals, and organizations aiming to strengthen healthcare, public health, veterinary medicine, agriculture, food safety, and research and manufacturing. Those goals include:

1) Slow the emergence of resistant bacteria and prevent the spread of resistant infections;
2) Strengthen national One-Health surveillance efforts to combat resistance;
3) Advance development and use of rapid and innovative diagnostic tests for identification and characterization of resistant bacteria;
4) Accelerate basic and applied research and development for new antibiotics, other therapeutics, and vaccines; and

5) Improve international collaboration and capacities for antibiotic-resistance prevention, surveillance, control, and antibiotic research and development

Taken together, implementation of specific objectives provided under each goal will help reduce the incidence of the priority pathogens listed in Table 1. National targets for reducing serious and urgent threats by 2020 are provided in Table 3.

Development and implementation of the *National Strategy* also supports World Health Assembly (WHA) resolution 67.25 (Antimicrobial Resistance), which was endorsed in May 2014 and urges countries to develop and finance national plans and strategies and take urgent action at the national, regional, and local levels to combat resistance. The resolution specifically calls on WHA Member States to develop practical and feasible approaches to extend the lifespan of drugs, strengthen pharmaceutical management systems and laboratory infrastructure, develop effective surveillance systems, and encourage the development of new diagnostics, drugs, and treatment options.

DEVELOPMENT OF THE STRATEGY

In December 2013, the President directed the National Security Council (NSC) and the Office of Science and Technology Policy (OSTP) to assess the current and growing threat of antibiotic resistance and develop a multi-sectoral plan to combat resistant bacteria. NSC and OSTP established an interagency policy committee to review past and current Federal efforts to address antibiotic resistance. The committee— which included representatives from the Department of Health and Human Services (HHS), the Department of Agriculture (USDA), the Departments of Homeland Security (DHS), State, Defense (DOD), Veterans Affairs (VA), the U.S. Agency for International Development (USAID), and the Environmental Protection Agency (EPA)— suggested practical, evidence-based ways to enhance antibiotic stewardship, strengthen surveillance for antibiotic resistance and use, advance the development of new diagnostics, antibiotics, and novel therapies, and accelerate research and innovation. The results of the review provided the basis for this *National Strategy*.

PARTNERSHIPS AND IMPLEMENTATION

The *National Strategy for Combating Antibiotic-Resistant Bacteria* will be implemented in accordance with a forthcoming *National Action Plan*, which will detail specific steps and milestones for achieving the *Strategy*'s goals and objectives along with metrics for measuring progress. The *National Action Plan* will also address recommendations made in the PCAST *Report to the President on Combating Antibiotic Resistance.*

Implementation of the *National Action Plan* will require the sustained, coordinated, and complementary efforts of individuals and groups around the world, including many who will contribute to its development. These include public and private sector partners, healthcare providers, healthcare leaders, veterinarians, agriculture industry leaders, manufacturers, policymakers, and patients. All of us who depend on antibiotics must join in a common effort to detect, stop, and prevent the emergence and spread of resistant bacteria.

GOAL 1: SLOW THE DEVELOPMENT OF RESISTANT BACTERIA AND PREVENT THE SPREAD OF RESISTANT INFECTIONS

The Opportunity

Judicious use of antibiotics is essential to slow the development of resistance, prevent outbreaks of untreatable infections, and extend the useful lifetime of our most urgently needed antibiotics. At the present time, however, one-third to one-half of all antibiotics used in inpatient and outpatient settings are either unnecessary or incorrectly prescribed.[2] The misuse and overuse of antibiotics not only facilitates the emergence of drug-resistant bacteria, but also exposes patients to needless risk for adverse effects.

Fortunately, a growing body of evidence demonstrates that programs dedicated to improving antibiotic use, known as "antibiotic stewardship" programs, can help slow the emergence of resistance while optimizing treatment and minimizing costs. These programs help providers prescribe the right antibiotic for the right amount of time and prevent prescription of antibiotics for non-bacterial infections. It is imperative that such programs become a routine and robust component of healthcare delivery in the United

States. To ensure success, improved data collection systems to monitor improvements in antibiotic usage must also be developed (*see also* Goal 2). Antibiotic stewardship is also needed in agricultural settings because bacteria associated with livestock may contribute to the development of resistance to drugs used in humans. In December 2013, the Food and Drug Administration (FDA) issued *Guidance for Industry* (GFI) #213,[3] which outlines voluntary measures to limit use of medically important antibiotics in livestock.

In addition to slowing the emergence of resistance, it is also critical to prevent transmission of bacteria-causing infections that are resistant to treatment across community and healthcare settings. Outbreaks can be prevented through regional efforts to rapidly detect and control infections that are hard to treat, and also through prompt communications regarding the management and transfer of infected patients within and between healthcare facilities. These interventions, which can be implemented nationally, will be supported by enhanced surveillance activities (Goal 2) that facilitate targeting the most important threats (see Table 1).

Objectives

1.1. Implement Public Health Programs and Reporting Policies That Advance Antibiotic-Resistance Prevention and Foster Antibiotic Stewardship in Healthcare Settings and the Community

Implementation steps include working with healthcare facilities, community and professional organizations, state and local health departments, and other partners to:

I. Strengthen antibiotic stewardship in inpatient, outpatient, and long-term care settings by expanding existing programs, developing new ones, and monitoring progress and efficacy. B. Strengthen educational programs such as *Get Smart: Know When Antibiotics Work*,[4] which inform physicians, agricultural workers, and members of the public about good antibiotic stewardship.

II. Expand collaborative efforts by groups of healthcare facilities that focus on preventing the spread of antibiotic resistant bacteria that pose a serious threat to public health (see Table 1).

III. Implement annual reporting of antibiotic use in inpatient and outpatient settings and identify geographic variations and/or variations at the provider and/or patient level that can help guide interventions.

IV. Develop and pilot new interventions to address geographic, socio-cultural, policy, economic, and clinical drivers of the emergence and spread of antibiotic resistance and misuse or over-use of antibiotics.

V. Streamline the regulatory processes for updating and approving antibiotic susceptibility testing devices, as appropriate, so that clinicians receive up-to-date interpretive criteria to guide antibacterial drug selection.

1.2. Eliminate the Use of Medically Important[5] Antibiotics for Growth Promotion in Animals and Bring Other In-Feed Uses of Antibiotics, for Treatment and Disease Control and Prevention of Disease, under Veterinary Oversight

Implementation steps include working with veterinary organizations, producers, producer organizations, the animal feed industry, the veterinary pharmaceutical industry, and other partners to:

I. Implement FDA Guidance for Industry #213 to eliminate the use of medically important antibiotics for growth promotion in animals and bring other therapeutic uses of medically important antibiotics under veterinary oversight. FDA should evaluate the adoption of the proposed changes under Guidance #213 during the three-year implementation period and take further action as appropriate.

II. Assess progress toward eliminating the use of medically important antibiotics for growth promotion in food-producing animals through enhanced data collection on antibiotic sales and use.

III. Develop and implement educational outreach efforts to ensure that veterinarians and animal producers receive information and training to support implementation of these changes.

IV. Optimize public awareness about the progress toward eliminating the use of medically important antibiotics for animal growth promotion.

1.3. Identify and Implement Measures to Foster Stewardship of Antibiotics in Animals

Implementation steps include working with veterinary organizations, animal producer organizations, and other partners to:

I. Develop, implement, and measure the effectiveness of evidence-based educational outreach to veterinarians and animal producers to advance antibiotic stewardship and judicious use of antibiotics in agricultural settings.

II. Foster collaborations and public-private partnerships with public health, pharmaceutical, and agricultural stakeholders to facilitate identification and implementation of interventions (e.g., good husbandry practices) to reduce the spread of antibiotic resistance.

III. Identify, develop, and revise key agricultural practices that allow timely and effective implementation of interventions that improve animal health and efficient production.

IV. Develop appropriate metrics to gauge the success of stewardship efforts and guide their continued evolution and optimization.

ANTICIPATED OUTCOMES

Federal agencies will meet these objectives in cooperation with the private sector and other stakeholders to meet the following benchmarks by 2020:

- All States, the District of Columbia, and Puerto Rico will have:
  - Implemented antibiotic stewardship activities in human healthcare delivery settings.
  - Established or enhanced regional efforts to reduce transmission of antibiotic-resistant pathogens and improve appropriate antibiotic use in healthcare facilities across the continuum of care (e.g., acute care, long term care, and outpatient care).
- HHS, DOD, and VA will review existing regulations and propose new regulations and other actions, as appropriate, which require hospitals and other inpatient healthcare delivery facilities to implement robust antibiotic stewardship programs that adhere to best practices, such as those defined by the CDC's Core Elements of Hospital Antibiotic Stewardship Programs.[6]
- At least 95% of eligible hospitals will report antibiotic use data to the National Healthcare Safety Network (NHSN).
- Inappropriate inpatient antibiotic use for monitored conditions/agents will be reduced by 20% from 2014 levels.
- Inappropriate outpatient antibiotic use for monitored conditions/agents will be reduced by 50% from 2010 levels.

- Eliminate the use of medically important antibiotics for growth promotion in animals.
- Use of medically important antibiotics in food-producing animals will require veterinary oversight.
- Research efforts will generate validated alternatives to traditional uses of antibiotics, such as changes to health and other management practices, to reduce the need for antibiotics for prevention and treatment of animal diseases.
- The Department of Health and Human Service's Agency for Healthcare Research & Quality and CDC will expand its focus on research and evaluation to develop improved methods and approaches for combating antibiotic resistance and conducting antibiotic stewardship.

GOAL 2: STRENGTHEN NATIONAL ONE-HEALTH SURVEILLANCE EFFORTS TO COMBAT RESISTANCE

The Opportunity

Collection and analysis of data on antibiotic resistance is an important component of biosurveillance, the process of "gathering, integrating, interpreting, and communicating essential information related to all-hazards threats or disease activity affecting human, animal, or plant health"[7] to improve outbreak detection and support decision-making. By linking human, animal, and plant health, this definition recognizes the importance of the *One-Health* approach to addressing emerging infectious diseases, an approach that emphasizes that the health of humans is connected to the health of animals and their shared environment.

Improved detection of resistant bacteria can be achieved through enhancements and expansion of existing surveillance systems that monitor resistance in healthcare settings (such as the National Healthcare Safety Network [NHSN]), in agricultural settings (such as the National Antimicrobial Resistance Monitoring System [NARMS]), and across healthcare and community settings (such as the Emerging Infections Program [EIP]). Enhancements include providing incentives for healthcare-facility reporting, advancing automatic capture of electronic data from healthcare facilities and clinical laboratories, including more diverse patient and community venues as reporting sites, and expanding the sampling of bacterial specimens from agricultural settings. Taken together, improvements to NHSN, EIP, and NARMS will enhance detection of emerging threats in humans and animals, speed outbreak response, and identify populations at greatest medical risk. Moreover, experience with NHSN has shown that reporting also leads to better prevention (Goal 1), because hospitals and state and local health departments use NHSN data to guide local action to interrupt the spread of resistant infections.

To be most useful, the data reported to these systems must be accurate and complete. For that reason, laboratories that test (and report on) resistant bacteria should be linked into a regional network that promotes the use of new technologies and diagnostics (see also Goal 3). The regional network will provide a standardized testing and reporting platform for antibiotic resistance, as well as advanced capacity for genetic characterization of bacteria with rare or unknown resistance mechanisms. These laboratories will serve as a resource that helps healthcare facilities and regional prevention programs investigate outbreaks, quantify the magnitude of resistance problems, and promote accurate testing practices at clinical laboratories. The laboratories that participate in the network will also help establish a national specimen repository for resistant bacteria and a national database of their DNA sequences.

Special investments are required to strengthen surveillance for antibiotic resistance among food animals and foods-of-animal-origin. Expanded capacity for testing, reporting, and data-sharing in veterinary and food safety laboratories will ensure early warning of the emergence of resistance in zoonotic and animal pathogens and enable officials to monitor the preventive impact of the FDA *Guidance for Industry* (GFI) #213 (see Goal 1). Efforts to monitor drug resistance patterns in food-producing animals, as well as collection of information on antibiotic drugs sold and distributed for use in food-producing animals, can build on or supplement NARMS, which tracks trends related to antibiotic resistance in food-producing animals, retail meats, and humans.

Objectives

2.1. Create a Regional Laboratory Network to Strengthen National Capacity to Detect Resistant Bacterial Strains and Create a Specimen Repository to Facilitate Development and Evaluation of Diagnostic Tests and Treatments

Implementation steps include working with healthcare facilities, state and local health departments, clinical laboratories, and many other partners to:

I. Create a regional laboratory network that uses standardized testing platforms to:
   - Expand the availability of reference testing services.
   - Characterize emerging resistance patterns and bacterial strains obtained from outbreaks and other sources.
   - Facilitate rapid data analysis and dissemination of information.

II. Link data generated by the regional laboratory network to:
   - Existing public health surveillance networks so that antimicrobial susceptibility testing (AST) data are immediately available to local, state and federal public health authorities as they detect and investigate outbreaks.
   - Veterinary diagnostic and food safety laboratory databases and/or surveillance systems, as needed.

III. Create a repository of resistant bacterial strains and maintain a well curated, reference database that describes the characteristics of these strains. The repository will aid:
   - Biotechnology and pharmaceutical companies that develop new antibiotics, therapeutics, and/or design next-generation tests for diagnosis and susceptibility testing.
   - Diagnostic test developers and regulatory agencies who evaluate these tests.
   - Government facilities, academic labs, and pharmaceutical companies that test antibiotics for clinical effectiveness.
   - Researchers, regulators, and others who assess the effectiveness of interventions to prevent resistance.
   - As part of these efforts, the Department of Defense will maintain a repository of resistant bacterial strains and, as appropriate, will update procedures for specimen collection, storage, and data-sharing.

IV. Develop and maintain a national sequence database of resistant pathogens.

2.2. Expand and Strengthen the National Infrastructure for Public Health Surveillance and Data Reporting and Provide Incentives for Timely Reporting of Antibiotic Resistance and Antibiotic Use in All Healthcare Settings

Implementation steps include working with governmental and non-governmental partners to:

I. Enhance reporting infrastructure and provide incentives for reporting (e.g., requiring reporting of antibiotic resistance data to NHSN as part of the Centers for Medicare and Medicaid [CMS] Hospital Inpatient Quality Reporting Program).
II. Add electronic reporting of antimicrobial use and resistance data in a standard file format to the Stage 3 Meaningful Use certification program for electronic health record systems.[8]
III. Expand the activities and scope of the Emerging Infections Program (EIP) to include monitoring additional urgent and serious bacterial threats (see Table 1) and evaluating populations at risk across community and healthcare settings.

2.3. Develop, Expand, and Maintain Capacity in State and Federal Veterinary and Food Safety Laboratories to Conduct Standardized Antibiotic Susceptibility Testing and Characterize Select Zoonotic and Animal Pathogens

Implementation steps include working with state and Federal veterinary and food safety laboratories and many other partners to:

I. Expand and maintain laboratory infrastructure for the identification of select zoonotic and animal health pathogens through the implementation of new diagnostic technologies (see also Goal 3).
II. Accelerate and standardize antibiotic susceptibility testing and bacterial characterization for select zoonotic and animal health pathogens, coordinating with appropriate stakeholder groups.
III. Enhance communications and identify mechanisms for sharing and reporting antibiotic susceptibility data on select zoonotic and animal

health pathogens collected by State and Federal veterinary diagnostic and food safety laboratories. These data should be stored in a centralized repository that can be linked with relevant public health databases, as appropriate, while maintaining source confidentiality.

2.4. Enhance Monitoring of Antibiotic-Resistance Patterns, as Well as Antibiotic Sales, Usage, and Management Practices, at Multiple Points in the Production Chain from Food-Animals On-Farm, Through Processing, and Retail Meat

Implementation steps include working with veterinary organizations, animal producer organizations, veterinary and food safety laboratories, and other partners to:

I. Enhance surveillance of antibiotic resistance in animal and zoonotic pathogens and commensal organisms by strengthening the National Antimicrobial Resistance Monitoring System (NARMS) and leveraging other field- and laboratory-based surveillance systems.
II. Enhance collection and reporting of data regarding antibiotic drugs sold and distributed for use in food-producing animals.
III. Implement voluntary monitoring of antibiotic use and resistance in pre-harvest settings to provide nationally-representative data while maintaining producer confidentiality.
IV. Collect quantitative data on antibiotic resistance and management practices along various points at pre-harvest, harvest, and processing, in collaboration with producers and other stakeholders and disseminate information as appropriate.

Anticipated Outcomes

In working towards these objectives with private sector and other stakeholders, Federal agencies will aim to meet the following milestones by 2020:

- Establishment of a regional laboratory network that conducts antibiotic susceptibility testing and other testing to identify outbreaks caused by antibiotic-resistant bacteria and to characterize emerging resistance patterns. The regional laboratory network will participate in international efforts to advance public health communications involving drug resistance (e.g., posting early warning alerts and reporting antibiotic resistance results and trends). See also Goal 5.3.

- Creation of a public electronic portal that will make antibiotic use and resistance data from CDC's monitoring systems publicly available, consistent with the Office Of Management and Budget's Open Data Policy (M 13-13).[9] Optimally, the portal should provide a unified, user-friendly database that facilitates integrated analyses of trends and practices at the state and regional levels.
- Creation of incentives for hospital reporting of data on antibiotic use and resistance to the NHSN, using the NHSN Antimicrobial Use and Resistance (AUR) Module[10] or equivalent update to achieve these reporting targets:
  - At least 95% of eligible hospitals report electronically captured antibiotic resistance data to NHSN.
  - 3,400 acute care hospitals using electronic health records that meet certification criteria for NHSN AUR reporting or successor standard as appropriate.
  - DOD and VA hospitals and long-term care facilities will also use electronic health records that meet certification criteria for AUR reporting or successor standard as appropriate.
- At least twenty veterinary diagnostic laboratories in the National Animal Health Laboratory Network and/or the Veterinary Laboratory Investigation and Response Network (Vet-LIRN) will routinely perform antibiotic susceptibility testing of bacterial strains for which standardized testing methods and data-sharing practices have been established.

GOAL 3: ADVANCE DEVELOPMENT AND USE OF RAPID AND INNOVATIVE DIAGNOSTIC TESTS FOR IDENTIFICATION AND CHARACTERIZATION OF RESISTANT BACTERIA

The Opportunity

Improved diagnostics for detection of resistant bacteria and characterization of their resistance patterns will help physicians make optimal treatment decisions and help public health officials take action to prevent and control disease.

Presently, most diagnostic tests take 24 to72 hours from specimen collection to results, with culture-based tests to determine antibiotic susceptibility adding additional days to weeks. Thus, treatment decisions are typically required and made before laboratory results are available. As a consequence, patients may be initially treated with antibiotics when none are needed, prescribed an inappropriate antibiotic, or treated with multiple antibiotics when a single antibiotic would have been effective.

However, the technological landscape is changing at a rapid pace. The current trend is moving towards clinical presentation or point-of-need diagnostic tests suitable for use during a healthcare visit because they require only minutes. In the future, widespread availability of point-of-need tests that rapidly distinguish between viral and bacterial infections will significantly reduce unnecessary antibiotic use. In addition, scientists will use knowledge of microbial genetics and the molecular determinants of antibiotic resistance to develop rapid, inexpensive molecular tests that identify not only an infecting pathogen, but also its antibiotic-resistance profile.

The development of rapid diagnostic tests, combined with ongoing use of culture-based tests to identify and investigate new resistance mechanisms, will greatly advance detection, control, and prevention of such threats as carbapenem-resistant Enterobacteriaceae (CRE), ceftriaxone resistant *N. gonorrhoeae*, Methicillin-resistant *Staphylococcus aureus* (MRSA), and other multidrug-resistant organisms (MDROs) (see Table 1). These tests will help guide outbreak responses, inform efforts to slow the development of resistance (e.g., the Antibiotic Stewardship programs described in Goal 2), and will have profound domestic and global utility.

In addition to supporting research on diagnostics (see Goal 4), the United States Government can help spur development of diagnostics by providing academic and private sector researchers with representative clinical isolates as well as the technical tools to help address issues related to test development and validation, FDA review, and reimbursement.

Objectives

3.1. Develop and Approve New Diagnostics, Including Tests That Rapidly Distinguish Between Viral and Bacterial Pathogens and Tests That Detect Antibiotic Resistance That Can Be Implemented in a Wide Range of Settings

United States Government departments and agencies will work with domestic and international partners to develop rapid diagnostic tests that can:

- Identify clinical illnesses that may benefit from treatment with antibiotics.
- Detect invasive bacterial pathogens in blood, cerebrospinal fluid, synovial fluid, and urine.
- Provide information to guide decisions on treatment and control of CRE, *Neisseria gonorrhoeae*, and other multidrug-resistant organisms.

3.2. Expand the Availability and Use of Diagnostics to Improve Treatment of Antibiotic-Resistant Bacteria, Enhance Infection Control, and Facilitate Outbreak Detection and Response in Healthcare and Community Settings

Anticipated Outcomes

In working toward these objectives with private sector and other stakeholders, Federal agencies will aim to meet the following benchmarks by 2020:

- Development and dissemination of licensed point-of-need diagnostic tests that distinguish between bacterial and viral infections in 20 minutes or less.
- Validation of diagnostic tests in late-stage clinical trials that determine antibiotic resistance profiles of the 18 bacteria of highest concern (Table 1) in 30 minutes or less.
- Development of well-defined reimbursement policies and incentives to encourage routine use of diagnostics in clinical settings to

distinguish between bacterial and viral infections and to ascertain the antibiotic susceptibilities of bacteria.

GOAL 4: ACCELERATE BASIC AND APPLIED RESEARCH AND DEVELOPMENT FOR NEW ANTIBIOTICS, OTHER THERAPEUTICS, AND VACCINES

The Opportunity

New therapeutics, vaccines, and diagnostics[11] are urgently needed to combat emerging and reemerging antibiotic-resistant pathogens. In response, the United States Government has accelerated efforts to advance the discovery and development of novel tools to address antibiotic resistance, with special attention to treatment of multidrug-resistant Gram-negative bacteria, such as CRE and *Neisseria gonorrhoeae,* which are of particular concern because of their diverse and rapidly evolving mechanisms of resistance.

Presently, the pipeline of antibiotics in development is inadequate and commercial interest in antibiotic development remains limited. Nevertheless, a cadre of dedicated innovators, many of them supported by Federal funds, are exploring ways to develop new classes of antibiotics as well as new therapies that could potentially replace the use of antibiotics in agriculture and humans. Efforts are focused at identifying and characterizing new drug targets and developing new therapeutic approaches.

Bringing promising antibiotic candidates to market is a major goal of the *Biomedical Advanced Research and Development Authority (BARDA),* which is working collaboratively with other government agencies to advance innovative research on antibiotic resistance. Examples include hosting research forums to facilitate the creation of public/private partnerships and launching a "biopharmaceutical incubator" that allows academic institutions and start-up companies to explore creative, early-stage research ideas that could lead to development of new antibacterial drugs or therapies.

Objectives

4.1. Conduct Research to Enhance Understanding of Environmental Factors That Facilitate the Development of Antibiotic Resistance and the Spread of Resistance Genes That Are Common to Animals and Humans

Implementation steps include working with academic and industry partners to:

I. Support basic research to utilize powerful new technologies and approaches including systems biology to advance the study of antibiotic resistance and address the special problems posed by resistant Gram-negative pathogens such as CRE.

II. Leverage existing partnerships, such as the Antibacterial Resistance Leadership Group (ARLG), to reduce obstacles faced by drug companies who are developing new antibiotics. For example, ARLG or another public-private partnership might:
   - Help identify human subjects qualified for enrollment in clinical trials of antibiotics to treat resistant bacterial infections that occur sporadically, episodically, and/or in limited populations.
   - Generate and apply common clinical test protocols to multiple test group of patients while sharing a common control group.

4.2. Increase Research Focused on Understanding the Nature of Microbial Communities, How Antibiotics Affect Them, and How They Can Be Harnessed to Prevent Disease

4.3. Intensify Research and Development of New Therapeutics and Vaccines, First-In-Class Drugs, and New Combination Therapies for Treatment of Bacterial Infections

4.4. Develop Non-Traditional Therapeutics and Innovative Strategies to Minimize Outbreaks Caused by Resistant Bacteria in Human and Animal Populations

4.5. Expand Ongoing Efforts to Provide Key Data and Materials to Support the Development of Promising Antibacterial Drug Candidates

4.6. Enhance Opportunities for Public-Private Partnerships to Accelerate Research on New Antibiotics and Other Tools to Combat Resistant Bacteria

4.7. Create a Biopharmaceutical Incubator—A Consortium of Academic, Biotechnology and Pharmaceutical Industry Partners—To Promote Innovation and Increase the Number of Antibiotics in the Drug-Development Pipeline

Anticipated Outcomes

In working toward these objectives with private sector and other stakeholders, Federal departments and agencies will aim to meet the following benchmarks by 2020:

- Two programs sponsored by BARDA will file FDA New Drug Applications for a new antibiotic by the end of 2018.
- Antibiotics developed by two other BARDA-sponsored programs will enter Phase III clinical development by the end of 2016.
- Antibiotics developed by DOD's Defense Threat Reduction Agency-sponsored program will submit pre-Emergency Use Authorization package in 2015.
- USDA will develop at least three drug candidates or probiotic treatments as alternatives to antibiotics for promoting growth in animals (see also Goal 1).
- FDA, USDA, CDC, and the National Institutes of Health (NIH) will encourage private-public sector partnerships to support antibiotic research by hosting a series of Round Table talks for experts in food production, agriculture, and public health.
- By the end of 2014, FDA, USDA, DHS, and National Science Foundation (NSF) will work with the National Institute for Mathematical and Biological Synthesis to develop an analytic modeling framework for assessing the relationship between antibiotic use in livestock (measured at the population level) and the development of antibiotic resistance. The framework will include early milestones and metrics for success.

- FDA, USDA, CDC, DOD and NIH will convene a joint summit to evaluate the status of ongoing research into mechanisms of resistance and its spread among zoonotic pathogens and commensal microbiota. The research projects may make use of whole genome sequencing, proteomics, metagenomics, structural biology, and bioinformatics.
- FDA, USDA, CDC, NIH, DOD, and EPA will conduct annual evaluations to ensure that research resources are focused on high-priority resistance issues.
- A mechanism will be in place to ensure that datasets on antibiotic resistance generated through federally funded research, including genomic and proteomic data sets, are publicly available through searchable online databases in a manner that is consistent with protecting personally identifiable information (see also Objective 2.1).
- The gut microbiome of at least one animal species raised for food will be sequenced and characterized to advance our understanding of the structure and function of gastrointestinal microbial communities. This research may help identify new growth promotants, antibacterial interventions that do not disrupt the normal gut intestinal microbiota of food animals, and may provide insight into management of the human microbiome.

GOAL 5 : IMPROVE INTERNATIONAL COLLABORATION AND CAPACITIES FOR ANTIBIOTIC RESISTANCE PREVENTION, SURVEILLANCE, CONTROL, AND ANTIBIOTIC RESEARCH AND DEVELOPMENT

The Opportunity

Domestic action alone is insufficient to protect the nation's public and agriculture health and security. Resistance occurs naturally, but careless practices in drug supply and use or overuse — both in the United States and in countries around the world - are rapidly increasing the prevalence of hard-to-treat infections in both animals and humans. Antibiotic resistance represents a major economic burden on healthcare systems as resistant strains of bacteria cost more to treat and often require prolonged treatment. In the worst of cases, a strain is resistant to all of the available drugs and presents a threat to our global health security. The pipeline for new and more effective antibiotics is not well-stocked, and without action, the world may soon lose the easiest way to treat infections and keep people alive and healthy.

Effectively combating antibiotic resistance will require government, industry, academia, and the human and animal health sectors across the globe to work together. The global community is faced with limited tools to address this global threat due to a critical lack of data on the magnitude, epidemiology and economic impact of antibiotic resistance, as well as the paucity of diagnostic and therapeutic options. The actions the United States takes domestically must be complemented by coordinated international action in order to ensure that resistant strains that arise in one part of the world are rapidly detected, diagnosed, and contained at the source of emergence. The United States and international partners must work to promote innovation in drug and diagnostics development, enhance stewardship of existing antibiotics in human and agricultural settings, and strengthen systems for detecting, diagnosing, and monitoring resistance so that reporting is timely, accurate, and transparent.

International momentum for addressing the urgent threat of antibiotic resistance continues to grow at a political level. The United States has supported ongoing exchanges with the European Union through the Trans-Atlantic Taskforce on Antimicrobial Resistance (TATFAR), which was established in 2009 by President Obama and his European counterparts to improve cooperation on combating resistance. TATFAR serves as an effective model for international collaboration on antibiotic resistance both in terms of enabling robust technical exchanges as well as facilitating transparency and identifying best practices. In June 2013, G8 Science Ministers collectively agreed that resistance is a “major health security challenge of the 21st century” and affirmed the pivotal role that science plays in addressing global challenges like drug resistance. Additionally, the recent endorsement of resolution 67.25 by the World Health Assembly has triggered an international, WHO-led process to develop a Global Action Plan for Antimicrobial Resistance. The United States continues vigorously to support this process, which will provide a broad framework that will facilitate coordinated national and global investments to combat resistance. The Global Health Security Agenda (GHSA), launched by the United States in partnership with nearly 30 countries in February 2014, includes preventing and detecting resistance as a key component, and the GHSA will provide an important forum for securing international financial and technical commitments to combat resistance in support of the WHO Global Action Plan.

United States Government agencies will work with ministries of health, agriculture, and food safety, WHO, Food and Animal Organization (FAO), World Organization for Animal Health (OIE), the European Union, and other partners to advance global efforts to combat antibiotic bacteria. Multilateral efforts will include: supporting the development of the WHO Global Action Plan to Address Antimicrobial Resistance; strengthening cooperation under the European Union-United States TATFAR; increasing political awareness regarding the health, economic, and security impacts of antibiotic resistance; and mobilizing broader international support to combat antibiotic resistance through venues such as the recently launched GHSA. As needed and appropriate, United States Government agencies will provide information, technical assistance, and/or capacity-building resources to underdeveloped and developing nations throughout the world.

Objectives

Surveillance: Establish capacity to detect, analyze, and report antibiotic resistance in order to make information needed for evidence-based decision making available in each country and globally.

5.1. Promote Laboratory Capability to Identify at Least Three of the Seven WHO Priority AMR Pathogens[12] Using Standardized, Reliable Detection Assays

The WHO AMR Pathogens and types of resistance of concern include:

- *Escherichia coli*: resistance to 3rd generation cephalosporins and to fluoroquinolones
- *Klebsiella pneumoniae*: resistance to 3rd generation cephalosporins and to carbapenems
- *Staphylococcus aureus*: methicillin resistance, or MRSA
- *Streptococcus pneumoniae*: resistance (non-susceptibility) to penicillin
- Non-Typhoidal *Salmonella* (NTS): resistance to fluoroquinolones
- *Shigella* species: resistance to fluoroquinolones
- *Neisseria gonorrhoeae*: reduced susceptibility to 3rd generation cephalosporins

5.2. Collaborate with WHO, OIE, and Other International Efforts Focused on the Development of Harmonized, Laboratory-Based Surveillance Capacity to Detect and Monitor Antibiotic Resistance in Relevant Animal and Foodborne Pathogens

5.3. Develop a Mechanism For International Communication of Critical Events That May Signify New Resistance Trends with Global Public and Animal Health Implications

5.4. Promote the Generation and Dissemination of Information Needed to Effectively Address Antibiotic Resistance By:

I. Supporting consistent international standards for determining whether bacteria are resistant to antibiotics.

II. Developing international collaborations to gather country-specific and regional information on drivers of antibiotic resistance, identify evidence-based interventions and adapt these strategies to new settings, and evaluate their effectiveness.

III. Provide technical assistance to developing nations to improve their capacity to detect and respond effectively to antibiotic resistance.

Research and Development: Incentivize development of therapeutics and diagnostics for humans and animals.

5.5. Establish and Promote International Collaboration and Public-Private Partnerships to Incentivize Development of New Therapeutics to Counter Antibiotic Resistance Including New, Next-Generation, and Other Alternatives to Antibiotics; Vaccines; and Affordable, Rapidly Deployable, Point-Of-Need Diagnostics

Prevention and Control: Strengthen systems in countries, regional networks, and global partnerships to prevent and control the emergence and spread of antibiotic resistance through evidence-based interventions, and monitor and evaluate the effectiveness of those interventions.

5.6. Support Countries to Develop and Implement National Plans to Combat Antibiotic Resistance and Strategies to Enhance Antimicrobial Stewardship

5.7. Partner with Other Nations to Promote Quality, Safety, and Efficacy of Antibiotics and Strengthen Their Pharmaceutical Supply Chains

5.8. Coordinate Regulatory Approaches by Collaborating with International Organizations Such as FAO and OIE to Harmonize International Data Submission Requirements and Risk Assessment Guidelines Related to the Licensure and/or Approval of Veterinary Medicinal Products Including Antibacterial Agents, Vaccines, and Diagnostics to the Extent Possible

Anticipated Outcomes

In working toward these objectives with private sector and other stakeholders, Federal agencies will aim to meet the following benchmarks by 2020:

- Work with at least 30 partner countries to develop surveillance capacity to monitor and slow the rate of increase of antibiotic resistance, including at least one reference laboratory per country capable of identifying at least three of the seven WHO priority AMR pathogens (see page 19) using standardized, reliable detection assays, and reporting these results appropriately.
- Work with international partners to support the development and implementation of the *WHO Global Action Plan for Antimicrobial Resistance (AMR).*
- Support the development of a secure website or portal for real-time data-sharing among international public health partners on antibiotic-resistant bacteria to facilitate early warning and notification of significant events to WHO, ECDC, and other relevant global public health organizations.
- Develop a common system with the European Union for sharing and analyzing bacterial resistance patterns for the 18 CDC priority

pathogens (Table 1), which include the seven WHO priority pathogens.

- Support efforts to harmonize and integrate antibiotic-resistance surveillance data on WHO and CDC priority pathogens generated by WHO regional surveillance networks.
- In collaboration with partner nations and the WHO, FAO, and OIE, explore the establishment of a common mechanism for accelerating investment in research on the development of new and next generation antibiotics, including novel therapeutics, vaccines, and rapid, inexpensive, and rapidly deployable, point-of-care diagnostics; similarly coordinate research on the microbiomes of various species of food animals.
- Forge key partnerships aimed at reducing the use of medically important antibiotics for growth promotion in food animals and strengthening antibiotic stewardship in all human settings.
- Collaborate with other OIE member countries to establish a global database to collect harmonized quantitative data on the use of antibacterial agents in animals.
- Establish a process for international communication of critical events that may signify new resistance trends, including those with global public health implications.
- Work with WHO, FAO, and OIE to build on Codex Alimentarius[13] and other risk-management frameworks to assess country-specific and regional drivers of antibiotic resistance and work with Ministries of Health and Agriculture to adopt interventions that have proven successful in other settings.

NEXT STEPS

Over the next six months, an interagency task force co-chaired by the Secretaries of Health and Human Services, Agriculture, and Defense will develop a National Action Plan for Combating Antibiotic-Resistant Bacteria that will detail the specific steps that agencies are taking, or will take, both individually and in coordination to implement this *National Strategy*. The task force will also address recommendations made in a recent report by the President's Council of Advisors on Science and Technology on Combating Antibiotic Resistance. The National Action Plan will establish clear milestones and metrics for success. These activities will be coordinated by the White House National Security Council and Office of Science and Technology Policy. Because this initiative will require a sustained effort, the task force will regularly report to the President on progress made in implementing the National Strategy and Action Plan, and toward achieving the National Targets described in Table 3. It is expected that departments and agencies would also take steps to combat antibiotic resistance that are not explicitly included in either the National Strategy or Action Plan; these efforts will also be included in the progress report to the President. Industry and other non-governmental organizations as well as international partners will play a key role in accelerating progress in combating antibiotic resistance. This *National Strategy* will solidify an ongoing partnership among these entities that will ensure resources are leveraged effectively to address this urgent threat to public health and national security.

The *National Strategy* is intended to promote greater investment and coordination of U.S. Government resources to reduce antibiotic-resistant bacteria, but the *National Strategy* is not a budget document and does not imply approval for any specific action under Executive Order 12866 or the Paperwork Reduction Act. The *National Strategy* will inform the Federal budget and regulatory development processes within the context of the goals articulated in the President's Budget. All activities included in the *National Strategy* are subject to budgetary constraints and other approvals, including the weighing of priorities and available resources by the Administration in formulating its annual budget and by Congress in legislating appropriations.

TABLE 1: CDC'S ANTIBIOTIC-RESISTANT THREATS IN THE UNITED STATES, 2013

URGENT Threat Level Pathogens

Clostridium difficile

- 250,000 infections per year requiring hospitalization or affecting hospitalized patients.
- 14,000 deaths per year.

- At least $1 billion in excess medical costs per year.
- *C. difficile* deaths increased 400% between 2000 and 2007 because of the emergence of a strain resistant to a common antibiotic class (fluoroquinolones).
- Almost half of infections occur in people younger than 65, but more than 90% of deaths occur in people 65 and older.
- Half of *C. difficile* infections first show symptoms in hospitalized or recently hospitalized patients, and half show symptoms in nursing-home patients or in people recently cared for in doctors' offices and clinics who received antibiotics.
- The majority (71%) of pediatric *Clostridium difficile* infections, which are bacterial infections that cause severe diarrhea and are potentially life-threatening, occur among children in the general community; 73 % were found to have recently taken antibiotics prescribed in doctor's offices for other outpatient settings.[14]

Carbapenem-Resistant *Enterobacteriaceae*

- Out of approximately 140,000 healthcare-associated *Enterobacteriaceae* infections per year, more than 9,000 are caused by CRE (7,900 CR-*Klebsiella* spp; 1,400 CR-*E. coli*).
- Over 600 deaths per year (520 CR-*Klebsiella* spp; 90 CR-*E. coli*).
- 44 states have had at least one type of CRE confirmed by CDC testing.
- CRE are resistant to nearly all antibiotics including carbapenems – an antibiotic of last resort.

Neisseria gonorrhoeae (Notifiable to CDC)

- *Neisseria gonorrhoeae* causes gonorrhea, is the second most common reportable infection in the United States, and is developing resistance to the cephalosporin antibiotics (such as ceftriaxone), the last-line effective treatment option for this infection.
- Of the 820,000 cases per year, 30% (246,000) now demonstrate resistance to at least one antibiotic.
- If ceftriaxone-resistant *N. gonorrhoeae* becomes widespread, the public health impact during a 10-year period is estimated to be 75,000 additional cases of pelvic inflammatory disease, 15,000 cases of

epididymitis, and 222 additional HIV infections, with an estimated direct medical cost of at least $235 million.

SERIOUS Threat Level Pathogens

Multidrug-Resistant *Acinetobacter*

- 12,000 healthcare-associated *Acinetobacter* infections occur in the U.S. of which 7,000 are multidrug-resistant.
- —500 deaths per year.
- At least three different classes of antibiotics no longer cure resistant *Acinetobacter* infections.

Drug-Resistant *Campylobacter*

- *Campylobacter* causes —1.3 Million infections, 13, 000 hospitalizations and 120 deaths each year; 310,000 (25%) drug-resistant *Campylobacter* infections are found each year.
- *Campylobacter* drug resistance increased from 13% in 1997 to 25% in 2011.
- *Campylobacter* spreads from animals to people through contaminated food, particularly raw or undercooked chicken and unpasteurized milk.
- Antibiotic use in food animals can and does result in resistant *Campylobacter* that can spread to humans.

Fluconazole-Resistant *Candida*

- Out of 46,000 Candida yeast infections per year, 3,400 (30%) of patients with bloodstream infections with DR-*Candida* die during their hospitalization.
- CDC estimates that each case of *Candida* infection results in 3-13 days of additional hospitalization and a total of $6,000-$29,000 in direct healthcare costs per patient.

Extended Spectrum 13-Lactamase (ESBL)-Producing *Enterbacteriaceae*

- Extended spectrum 13-lactamase (ESBL) is an enzyme that makes bacteria resistant to a wide spectrum of penicillins and cephalosporins.
- Of 140,000 *Enterobacteriaceae* infections per year, 26,000 are drug-resistant, causing 1,700 deaths.
- 26,000 healthcare-associated *Enterobacteriaceae* infections are caused by ESBL- *Enterobacteriaceae.*
- *Enterobacteriaceae* infections result in greater than $40,000 excess hospital charges per occurrence.

Vancomycin-Resistant *Enterococcus*

- Of 66,000 *Enterococcus* infections per year, 20,000 are drug-resistant causing 1,300 deaths.

Enterococcus strains resistant to vancomycin have few or no treatment options. Multidrug-Resistant *Pseudomonas aeruginosa*

- Of 51,000 *Pseudomonas* infections per year, 6,700 are multidrug-resistant causing 440 deaths.
- 13% of severe healthcare-associated infections caused by *Pseudomonas* are multidrug resistant, meaning nearly all or all antibiotics no longer cure these infections.

Drug-Resistant Non-Typhoidal *Salmonella* (Notifiable to CDC)

- Non-typhoidal *Salmonella* causes 1.2 million infections per year, of which 100,000 are drug-resistant resulting in 23,000 hospitalizations and 450 deaths each year.
- Non-typhoidal *Salmonella* results in more hospitalizations, longer stays, and higher treatment costs.

Drug-Resistant *Salmonella enterica serovar Typhi* (Notifiable to CDC)

- Of 21.7 M *Salmonella typhi* infections worldwide, 5,700 illnesses in the U.S. with 3,800 (67%) of infections are drug-resistant resulting in 620 hospitalizations each year.
- Before the antibiotic era or in areas where antibiotics are unavailable, 20% of *Salmonella typhi* infections result in death.

Drug-Resistant *Shigella* (Notifiable to CDC)

- *Shigella* causes ~500,000 illnesses, 5,500 hospitalizations, and 40 deaths each year in the U.S.
- Since 2006, *Shigella* resistance to traditional first-line antibiotics has become so high that physicians must now rely on alternative drugs (ciprofloxacin and azithromycin) to treat infections.

Methicillin-Resistant *Staphylococcus aureus* (MRSA)

- Over 80,000 invasive MRSA infections and 11,285 related deaths per year (in 2011).
- Severe MRSA infections most commonly occur during or soon after inpatient medical care.
- Between 2005 and 2001, overall rates of invasive MRSA dropped 31% predominantly due to appropriate medical procedures implemented in central-line maintenance.

Drug-Resistant *Streptococcus pneumoniae* (Notifiable to CDC)

- Of 4 million disease incidents and 22,000 deaths, 1.2 M are drug-resistant [to amoxicillin and azithromycin (Z-Pak)], resulting in 19,000 excess hospitalizations and 7,900 deaths.
- In 30% of *S. pneumoniae* cases, the bacteria are fully resistant to one or more antibiotics, causing complications in treatment and death.
- Pneumococcal pneumonia accounts for 72% of all direct medical costs for treatment of pneumococcal disease and in excess of $96 million in medical costs per year.

- Pneumococcal conjugate vaccine (PCV) prevents disease, reduces antibiotic resistance by blocking the transmission of resistant *S. pneumoniae* strains, and protects against 13 strains of *S. pneumoniae*.

Drug-Resistant *Tuberculosis* (Notifiable to CDC)

- Tuberculosis (TB) is among the most common infectious diseases and cause of death worldwide.
- Of 9,588 TB cases in the U.S. in 2013, it is estimated that 1-2% of these cases were resistant to antibiotics with direct costs for treatment of MDR-TB averaging $134,000 per case (in 2010 dollars).
- CDC funds health departments in all 50 states, 10 large cities, DC, Puerto Rico, the Virgin Islands and other territories to conduct surveillance, provide laboratory testing, perform contact investigations, diagnose cases and provide directly-observed therapy and medical management for TB cases and therapy for latent TB infection. Five TB Regional Training and Medical Consultation Centers (RTMCCs) provide training and medical consultation for these programs.

OF CONCERN Threat Level Pathogens

Vancomycin-Resistant *Staphylococcus aureus* (Notifiable to CDC)

- Few cases, thus far (13 cases in 4 States since 2002).
- Staph *aureus* strains resistant to vancomycin have very few or no treatment options. Erythromycin-Resistant Group A *Streptococcus*
- Group A Strep (GAS) causes many illnesses, including strep throat (up to 2.6 M cases per year), toxic shock syndrome, and "flesh-eating" disease (necrotizing fasciitis, 25-35% fatal).
- Erythromycin-resistant GAS causes 1,300 illnesses and 160 deaths.
- Current concern is the increase in bacteria that show resistance to clindamycin, which has a unique role in treatment of GAS infections.

Clindamycin-Resistant Group B *Streptococcus*

- Of 27,000 GBS cases, 7,600 illnesses are drug-resistant, resulting in 440 deaths in the United States each year.

Additional information may be found in the CDC report *Antibiotic* resistance threats in the United States, 2013 (http://www.cdc.gov/drugresistance/threat-report-2013/).

TABLE 2: GOALS AND OBJECTIVES FOR COMBATING ANTIBIOTIC-RESISTANT BACTERIA

Goal 1: Slow the Emergence of Resistant Bacteria and Prevent the Spread of Resistant Infections

Objectives

1.1. Implement public health programs and reporting policies that advance antibiotic-resistance prevention and foster antibiotic stewardship in healthcare settings and the community.

1.2. Eliminate the use of medically important antibiotics for growth promotion in animals and bring other in-feed uses of antibiotics, for treatment and disease control and prevention of disease, under veterinary oversight.

1.3. Identify and implement measures to foster stewardship of antibiotics in animals.

Goal 2: Strengthen National One-Health Surveillance Efforts to Combat Resistance

Objectives

2.1. Create a regional laboratory network to strengthen national capacity to detect resistant bacterial strains and a specimen repository to facilitate development and evaluation of diagnostic tests and treatments.

2.2. Expand and strengthen the national infrastructure for public health surveillance and data reporting, and provide incentives for timely reporting of antibiotic resistance and antibiotic use in all healthcare settings.

2.3. Develop, expand, and maintain capacity in State and Federal veterinary and food safety laboratories to conduct standardized antibiotic susceptibility testing and characterize select zoonotic and animal pathogens.

2.4. Enhance monitoring of antibiotic-resistance patterns, as well as antibiotic sales, usage, and management practices, at multiple points in the production chain from food-animals on-farm, through processing, and retail meat.

Goal 3. Advance Development and Use of Rapid and Innovative Diagnostic Tests for Identification and Characterization of Resistant Bacteria

Objectives

3.1. Develop and approve new diagnostics, including tests that rapidly distinguish between viral and bacterial pathogens and tests that detect antibiotic resistance that can be implemented easily in a wide range of settings.

3.2. Expand availability and use of diagnostics to improve treatment of antibiotic-resistant infections, enhance infection control, and facilitate outbreak detection and response in healthcare and community settings.

Goal 4: Accelerate Basic and Applied Research and Development for New Antibiotics, Other Therapeutics, and Vaccines

Objectives

4.1. Conduct research to enhance understanding of ecological determinants and environmental factors that facilitate the development of antibiotic resistance and the spread of resistance genes that are common to animals and humans.

4.2. Increase research focused on understanding the nature of microbial communities, how antibiotics affect them, and how they can be harnessed to prevent disease.

4.3. Intensify research and development of new therapeutics and vaccines, first-in-class drugs, and new combination therapies for treatment of bacterial infections.

4.4. Develop non-traditional therapeutics and innovative strategies to minimize the effects of resistant bacteria in human and animal populations.

4.5. Expand ongoing efforts to provide key data and materials to support the development of promising antibacterial candidates.

4.6. Enhance opportunities for public-private partnerships to accelerate research on new antibiotics and other tools to combat resistant bacteria.

4.7. Create a biopharmaceutical incubator—a consortium of academic, biotechnology and pharmaceutical industry partners—to promote innovation and increase the number of antibiotics in the drug-development pipeline.

Goal 5: Improve International Collaboration and Capacities for Antibiotic Resistance Prevention, Surveillance, Control, and Antibiotic Research and Development

Objectives

Surveillance for Resistant Bacteria

5.1. Promote laboratory capability to identify at least 3 of the 7 WHO priority AMR pathogens[15] using standardized, reliable detection assays.

5.2. Collaborate with WHO, OIE, and other international efforts focused on the development of harmonized, laboratory-based surveillance capacity to detect and monitor antibiotic resistance in relevant animal and foodborne pathogens.

5.3. Develop a mechanism for international communication of critical events that may signify new resistance trends with global public and animal health implications.

5.4. Promote the generation and dissemination of information needed to address antibiotic resistance by:

5.4.1. Promote consistent international standards for determining whether bacteria are resistant to antibiotics; and

a) Develop international collaborations to gather country-specific and regional information on drivers of antibiotic resistance, identify evidence-based interventions, adapt these strategies to new settings, and evaluate their effectiveness; and
b) Provide technical assistance as needed to underdeveloped and developing nations to improve their capacity to detect and respond effectively to antibiotic resistance.

Research and Development

5.5.Establish and promote international collaboration and public-private partnerships to incentivize development of new therapeutics to counter antibiotic resistance including new, next-generation, and other alternatives to antibiotics; vaccines; and affordable, rapidly deployable, point-of-need diagnostics.

Prevention and Control

5.6. Support countries to develop and implement national plans to combat antibiotic resistance and strategies to enhance antimicrobial stewardship.

5.7. Partner with other nations to promote quality, safety, and efficacy of antibiotics and strengthen country pharmaceutical supply chains.

5.8. Coordinate regulatory approaches by collaborating with international organizations such as FAO and OIE to harmonize international data submission requirements and risk assessment guidelines related to the licensure and/or approval of veterinary medicinal products including antibiotics, vaccines, and diagnostics, to the extent possible.

TABLE 3: NATIONAL TARGETS FOR COMBATING ANTIBIOTIC-RESISTANT BACTERIA

By 2020, the United States will:

For CDC Recognized Urgent Threats:

- Reduce by 50% the incidence of overall *Clostridium difficile* infection compared to estimates from 2011.
- Reduce by 60% carbapenem-resistant *Enterobacteriaceae* infections acquired during hospitalization compared to estimates from 2011.
- Maintain the prevalence of ceftriaxone-resistant *Neisseria gonorrhoeae* below 2% compared to estimates from 2013.

For CDC Recognized Serious Threats:

- Reduce by 35% multidrug-resistant *Pseudomonas* spp. infections acquired during hospitalization compared to estimates from 2011.
- Reduce by at least 50% overall methicillin-resistant *Staphylococcus aureus* (MRSA) bloodstream infections by 2020 as compared to 2011.*

- Reduce by 25% multidrug-resistant non-typhoidal *Salmonella* infections compared to estimates from 2010—2012.
- Reduce by 15% the number of multidrug-resistant TB infections.
- Reduce by at least 25% the rate of antibiotic-resistant invasive pneumococcal disease among <5 year-olds compared to estimates from 2008.
- Reduce by at least 25%the rate of antibiotic-resistant invasive pneumococcal disease among >65 year-olds compared to estimates from 2008.

* This target is consistent with the reduction goal for MRSA bloodstream infections (BSI) in the *National Action Plan to Prevent Healthcare-Associated Infections (HAI): Road Map to Elimination,* which calls for a 75% decline in MRSA BSI from the 2007-2008 baseline by 2020. Additional information is available at http://www.health.gov/hai/prevent hai.asp#hai plan.

End Notes

[1] Centers for Disease Control and Prevention. Antibiotic Resistance Threats in the United States, 2013 (http://www.cdc.gov/drugresistance/threat-report-2013/)

[2] Centers for Disease Control and Prevention. Antibiotic Resistance Threats in the United States, 2013 (http://www.cdc.gov/drugresistance/threat-report-2013/); and Vital Signs: Improving Antibiotic Use Among Hospitalized Patients. MMWR March 7, 2014 / 63(09); 194-200.

[3] FDA Guidance for Industry #213 may be accessed at: http://www.fda.gov/downloads/animalveterinary/guidancecomplianceenforcement/guidanceforindustry/ucm299624.pdf.

[4] Examples of educational programs on antibiotic stewardship include: Get Smart: Know When Antibiotics Work (www.cdc.gov/getsmart); Get Smart for Healthcare (http://www.cdc.gov/getsmart/healthcare/index.html); and Get Smart: Know When Antibiotics Work on the Farm (http://www.cdc.gov/narms/get-smart.html).

[5] http://www.fda.gov/downloads/AnimalVeterinary/GuidanceComplianceEnforcement/GuidanceforIndustry /UCM299624.pdf (p. 5).

[6] The CDC's Core Elements of Hospital Antibiotic Stewardship Programs may be accessed at: http://www.cdc.gov/getsmart/healthcare/implementation/core-elements.html.

[7] See: http://www.whitehouse.gov/sites/default/files/National Strategy for Biosurveillance July 2012. pdf.

[8] Information on the CMS Meaningful Use program is available at: http://www.cms.gov/Regulations-andGuidance/Legislation/EHRIncentive Programs/ Meaningful Use.html.

[9] http://www.whitehouse.gov/sites/default/files/omb/memoranda/2013/m-13-13.pdf.

[10] Information on the NHSN Antimicrobial Use and Resistance (AUR) Module is available at: http://www.cdc.gov/nhsn/PDFs/pscManual/11pscAURcurrent.pdf.

[11] Diagnostics development is also discussed in Goal 2.

[12] The WHO priority AMR pathogens are a subset of the pathogens identified as urgent and serious threats in Table 1.

[13] The Codex Alimentarius is a collection of internationally recognized standards, codes of practice, and guidelines relating to foods, food production, and food safety (http://www.codexalimentarius.org/codexhome/en/).

[14] Wendt, J.M. et al. Clostridium difficile Infection Among Children Across Diverse US Geographic Locations. Pediatrics. January 3, 2014.

[15] A list of WHO priority AMR pathogens is provided on page 18. These pathogens are a subset of the pathogens identified as Urgent and Serious Threats in Table 1.

In: National Strategy
Editor: Anthony Phillips

ISBN: 978-1-63483-072-0

Chapter 2

NATIONAL ACTION PLAN FOR COMBATING ANTIBIOTIC-RESISTANT BACTERIA*

Task Force for Combating Antibiotic-Resistant Bacteria

EXECUTIVE SUMMARY

Antibiotics have been a critical public health tool since the discovery of penicillin in 1928, saving the lives of millions of people around the world. Today, however, the emergence of drug resistance in bacteria is reversing the miracles of the past eighty years, with drug choices for the treatment of many bacterial infections becoming increasingly limited, expensive, and, in some cases, nonexistent. The Centers for Disease Control and Prevention (CDC) estimates that drug-resistant bacteria cause two million illnesses and approximately 23,000 deaths each year in the United States alone.

The *National Action Plan for Combating Antibiotic-resistant Bacteria* provides a roadmap to guide the Nation in rising to this challenge. Developed in response to Executive Order 13676: Combating Antibiotic-Resistant Bacteria—issued by President Barack Obama on September 18, 2014—the *National Action Plan* outlines steps for implementing the *National Strategy for Combating Antibiotic-Resistant Bacteria* and addressing the policy recommendations of the President's Council of Advisors on Science and Technology (PCAST). Although its primary purpose is to guide activities by

---

* This is an edited, reformatted and augmented version of a document issued by the Executive Office of the President, March 2015.

the U.S. Government, the *National Action Plan* is also designed to guide action by public health, healthcare, and veterinary partners in a common effort to address urgent and serious drug-resistant threats that affect people in the U.S. and around the world. Implementation of the National Action Plan will also support World Health Assembly resolution 67.25 (Antimicrobial Resistance), which urges countries to take urgent action at the national, regional, and local levels to combat resistance.

The Goals of the *National Action Plan* Include

1) Slow the Emergence of Resistant Bacteria and Prevent the Spread of Resistant Infections.
2) Strengthen National One-Health Surveillance Efforts to Combat Resistance.
3) Advance Development and Use of Rapid and Innovative Diagnostic Tests for Identification and Characterization of Resistant Bacteria.
4) Accelerate Basic and Applied Research and Development for New Antibiotics, Other Therapeutics, and Vaccines.
5) Improve International Collaboration and Capacities for Antibiotic-resistance Prevention, Surveillance, Control, and Antibiotic Research and Development.

By 2020, implementation of the *National Action Plan* will lead to major reductions in the incidence of urgent and serious threats, including carbapenem-resistant *Enterobacteriaceae* (CRE), methicillin resistant *Staphylococcus aureus* (MRSA), and *Clostridium difficile* (see Table 1). The *National Action Plan* will also result in improved antibiotic stewardship in healthcare settings, prevention of the spread of drug-resistant threats, elimination of the use of medically-important antibiotics for growth promotion in food animals, and expanded surveillance for drug-resistant bacteria in humans and animals. Other significant outcomes include creation of a regional public health laboratory network, establishment of a specimen repository and sequence database that can be accessed by industrial and academic researchers, development of new diagnostic tests through a national challenge, and development of two or more antibiotic drug candidates or non-traditional therapeutics for treatment of human disease. In addition, the effort to combat resistant bacteria will become an international priority for global health security.

Progress towards achieving these outcomes will be monitored by the U.S. Government Task Force that developed the *National Action Plan.* The Task Force, which is co-chaired by the Secretaries of Defense, Agriculture, and Health and Human Services, includes representatives from the Departments of State, Justice, Veterans Affairs, and Homeland Security, as well as the Environmental Protection Agency, the United States Agency for International Development, the Office of Management and Budget, the Domestic Policy Council, the National Security Council, the Office of Science and Technology Policy, and the National Science Foundation. Additionally, the Presidential Advisory Council on Combating Antibiotic-Resistant Bacteria, created by Executive Order 13676, will provide advice, information, and recommendations to the Secretary of Health and Human Services regarding the *National Action Plan's* programs and policies and their impact on the threat.

Implementation of the objectives and activities in the *National Action Plan* requires sustained, coordinated, and complementary efforts of individuals and groups around the world, including healthcare providers, healthcare leaders, veterinarians, agriculture industry leaders, manufacturers, policymakers, and patients. All of us who depend on antibiotics must join in a common effort to detect, stop, and prevent the emergence and spread of resistant bacteria.

INTRODUCTION

> *Vision:* The United States will work domestically and internationally to prevent, detect, and control illness and death related to infections caused by antibiotic-resistant bacteria by implementing measures to mitigate the emergence and spread of antibiotic-resistance and ensuring the continued availability of therapeutics for the treatment of bacterial infections.

Antibiotics have been a critical public health tool since the discovery of penicillin in 1928, saving the lives of millions of people around the world. Today, however, the emergence of drug resistance in bacteria is reversing the gains of the past eighty years, with many important drug choices for the treatment of bacterial infections becoming increasingly limited, expensive, and, in some cases, nonexistent. The Centers for Disease Control and

Prevention (CDC) estimates that each year at least two million illnesses and 23,000 deaths are caused by drug-resistant bacteria in the United States alone.

The loss of antibiotics that kill or inhibit the growth of bacteria means that we can no longer take for granted quick and reliable treatment of rare or common bacterial infections, including bacterial pneumonias, foodborne illnesses, and healthcare-associated infections. As more strains of bacteria become resistant to an ever larger number of antibiotics, we will also lose the benefits of a range of modern medical procedures—from hip replacements to organ transplants—whose safety depends on our ability to treat bacterial infections that may arise as post-surgical complications. Moreover, antibiotic-resistance also threatens animal health, agriculture, and the economy.

The *National Action Plan for Combating Antibiotic-resistant Bacteria* provides a roadmap to guide the Nation in rising to this challenge. The *National Action Plan* outlines steps for implementing the *National Strategy for Combating Antibiotic-Resistant Bacteria* and addressing the policy recommendations of the President's Council of Advisors on Science and Technology. Although its primary purpose is to guide activities by the U.S. Government, the *National Action Plan* is also designed to guide action by public health, healthcare, and veterinary partners in a common effort to address urgent and serious drug-resistant threats (Table 3) that affect people in the U.S. and around the world.

Scope of the *National Action Plan:* "Antibiotic resistance" results from mutations or acquisition of new genes in bacteria that reduce or eliminate the effectiveness of antibiotics. "Antimicrobial resistance" is a broader term that encompasses resistance to drugs to treat infections caused by many different types of pathogens, including bacteria, viruses (e.g., influenza and the human immunodeficiency virus (HIV)), parasites (e.g., the parasitic protozoan that causes malaria), and fungi (e.g., *Candida spp.*). While all of these pathogens are dangerous to human health, the *National Action Plan* focuses on resistance in bacteria that present an urgent or serious threat to public health.

Goals of the National Action Plan

The *National Action Plan*—informed by the guiding principles in Table 2—is organized around five goals for collaborative action by the U.S. Government, in partnership with foreign governments, individuals, and organizations aiming to strengthen healthcare, public health, veterinary medicine, agriculture, food safety, and research and manufacturing. Aggressive action will move the nation towards major reductions in the incidence of urgent and serious drug-resistant threats (Table 3), including carbapenem resistant *Enterobacteriaceae* (CRE), methicillin-resistant *Staphylococcus aureus* (MRSA), and *Clostridium difficile.*

- Misuse and over-use of antibiotics in healthcare and food production continue to hasten the development of bacterial drug resistance, leading to loss of efficacy of existing antibiotics.
- Detecting and controlling antibiotic-resistance requires the adoption of a "One-Health" approach to disease surveillance that recognizes that resistance can arise in humans, animals, and the environment.
- Implementation of evidence-based infection control practices can prevent the spread of resistant pathogens.
- Interventions are necessary to accelerate private sector investment in the development of therapeutics to treat bacterial infections because current private sector interest in antibiotic development is limited.
- Researchers can use innovations and new technologies—including whole genome sequencing, metagenomics, and bioinformatic approaches—to develop next-generation tools to strengthen human and animal health, including:
    - Point-of-need diagnostic tests to distinguish rapidly between bacterial and viral infections as well as identify bacterial drug susceptibilities;
    - New antibiotics and other therapies that provide much needed treatment options for those infected with resistant bacterial strains; and
    - Antibiotic resistance is a global health problem that requires international attention and collaboration, because bacteria do not recognize borders.

Table 1. National Targets to Combat Antibiotic-Resistant Bacteria

By 2020, the United States will:
For CDC Recognized Urgent Threats:
Reduce by 50% the incidence of overall Clostridium difficile infection compared to estimates from 2011

Table 1. (Continued)

Reduce by 60% carbapenem-resistant Enterobacteriaceae infections acquired during hospitalization compared to estimates
Maintain the prevalence of ceftriaxone-resistant Neisseria gonorrhoeae below 2% compared to estimates from 2013
For CDC Recognized Serious Threats:
Reduce by 35% multidrug-resistant Pseudomonas spp infections acquired during hospitalization compared to estimates from 2011
Reduce by at least 50% overall methicillin-resistant Staphylococcus aureus (MRSA) bloodstream infections by 2020 as compared to 2011 *
Reduce by 25% multidrug-resistant non-typhoidal Salmonella infections compared to estimates from 2010-2012
Reduce by 15% the number of multidrug-resistant TB infections[1]
Reduce by at least 25% the rate of antibiotic-resistant invasive pneumococcal disease among <5 year-olds compared to estimates from 2008
Reduce by at least 25%the rate of antibiotic-resistant invasive pneumococcal disease among >65 year-olds compared to estimates from 2008

* This target is consistent with the reduction goal for MRSA bloodstream infections (BSI) in the *National Action Plan to Prevent Healthcare-Associated Infections (HAI): Road Map to Elimination,* which calls for a 75% decline in MRSA BSI from the 2007-2008 baseline by 2020. Additional information is available at http://www.health hai.asp#hai plan.

Those goals include:

GOAL 1: Slow the Emergence of Resistant Bacteria and Prevent the Spread of Resistant Infections. Judicious use of antibiotics in healthcare and agricultural settings is essential to slow the emergence of resistance and extend the useful lifetime of effective antibiotics. Antibiotics are a precious resource, and preserving their usefulness will require cooperation and engagement by healthcare providers, healthcare leaders, pharmaceutical companies, veterinarians, the agricultural industry, and patients. Goal 1 activities include the optimal use of vaccines to prevent infections, implementation of healthcare policies and antibiotic stewardship programs that improve patient outcomes, and efforts to minimize the development of resistance by ensuring that each patient receives *the right antibiotic at the right time at the right dose for the right duration.* Prevention of resistance also requires rapid detection and control of outbreaks and regional efforts to control transmission across community and healthcare settings.

GOAL 2: Strengthen National One-Health Surveillance Efforts to Combat Resistance. Improved detection and control of drug-resistant organisms will be achieved through an integrated, "One-Health" approach that includes the enhancement and integration of data from surveillance systems that monitor human pathogens—including the National Healthcare Safety Network (NHSN), the Emerging Infections Program (EIP), and the National Antimicrobial Resistance Monitoring System (NARMS)—with data from surveillance systems that monitor animal pathogens—including the National Animal Health Monitoring System (NAHMS), the National Animal Health Laboratory Network (NAHLN), and the Veterinary Laboratory Investigation and Response Network (Vet-LIRN). Goal 2 activities include creation of a regional public health laboratory network that provides a standardized platform for resistance testing and advanced capacity for genetic characterization of bacteria (e.g., through whole genome sequencing). Goal 2 activities will also enhance monitoring of antibiotic sales, usage, resistance, and management practices at multiple points along in the food-production chain, from farms to processing plants to supermarkets.

GOAL 3: Advance Development and Use of Rapid and Innovative Diagnostic Tests for Identification and Characterization of Resistant Bacteria. Improved diagnostics for detection of resistant bacteria and characterization of resistance patterns will help healthcare providers make optimal treatment decisions and assist public health officials in taking action to prevent and control disease. Improved diagnostics will also help decrease unnecessary or inappropriate use of antibiotics. Goal 3 activities will accelerate the development of new diagnostics and expand their availability and use to improve treatment, enhance infection control, and achieve faster response to infections and outbreaks caused by resistant bacteria in hospitals and in the community.

GOAL 4: Accelerate Basic and Applied Research and Development for New Antibiotics, Other Therapeutics, and Vaccines. Despite the urgent need for new antibiotics, the number of products in the drug-development pipeline is small and commercial interest remains limited. The advancement of drug development—as well as non-traditional therapeutics and vaccines—will require intensified efforts to boost scientific research, attract private investment, and facilitate clinical trials of new drug candidates. Goal 4 activities will help accomplish these objectives by supporting basic and applied research, providing researchers with scientific services (e.g., specimens, sequence data, and regulatory guidance), and fostering public-private partnerships that strengthen the clinical trials infrastructure and reduce the risks, uncertainty, and obstacles faced by companies who are developing new antibiotics and/or other therapeutics and vaccines that can impact the use of antibiotics and the development of resistance.

GOAL 5: Improve International Collaboration and Capacities for Antibiotic-resistance Prevention, Surveillance, Control, and Antibiotic Research and Development. Antibiotic resistance is a worldwide problem that cannot be addressed by one nation in isolation. Goal 5 activities include working with foreign ministries of health and agriculture, the World Health Organization (WHO), the Food and Agriculture Organization (FAO), the World Organization for Animal Health (OIE), and other multinational organizations to enhance global capacity to detect, analyze, and report antibiotic use and resistance, create incentives for the development of therapeutics and diagnostics, and strengthen global efforts to prevent and control the emergence and spread of antibiotic-resistance. To advance these objectives, U.S. agencies will support development of a *WHO Global Action Plan on Antimicrobial Resistance*, enhance international collaborations including cooperation under the European Union-United States Trans-Atlantic Task Force on Antimicrobial Resistance (TATFAR), and mobilize global health resources through the Global Health Security Agenda.

Development of the National Action Plan

The *National Action Plan* was developed in response to Executive Order 13676: Combating Antibiotic-Resistant Bacteria (Appendix 2), which was issued by President Barack Obama on September 18, 2014 in conjunction with the *National Strategy for Combating Antibiotic-Resistant Bacteria.*

The Executive Order calls for a U.S. Government Task Force to create a five-year action plan that lays out steps and milestones for achieving the *Strategy's* goals and objectives (Table 2) and addressing the PCAST recommendations. The Task Force, which is co-chaired by the Secretaries of Defense, Agriculture, and Health and Human Services, includes representatives from the Department of State, the Department of Justice, the Department of Veterans Affairs, the Department of Homeland Security, the

Environmental Protection Agency, the United States Agency for International Development, the Office of Management and Budget, the Domestic Policy Council, the National Security Council staff, the Office of Science and Technology Policy, and the National Science Foundation.

Development of the *National Action Plan* also supports World Health Assembly (WHA) resolution 67.25 (Antimicrobial Resistance), which was endorsed in May 2014 and urges countries to develop and finance national plans and strategies and take urgent action at the national, regional, and local levels to combat resistance. The resolution urges WHA Member States to develop practical and feasible approaches to, among other actions, extend the lifespan of drugs, strengthen pharmaceutical management systems and laboratory infrastructure, develop effective surveillance systems, and encourage the development of new diagnostics, drugs, and treatment options.

These recommendations are intended to inform the policy development process, and are not intended as a budget document. The commitment of resources to support these activities will be determined through the usual Executive Branch budget processes. Implementation of some of the actions in this report will require additional resources and these resources could be new or redirected from lower-priority Agency activities.

Monitoring and Evaluation

The Task Force created under Executive Order 13676 is charged with providing the President with annual updates on Federal Government actions to combat antibiotic resistance, including progress made in implementing the *National Action Plan*, plans for addressing obstacles and challenges, and recommendations for new or modified actions. The Presidential Advisory Council on Combating Antibiotic-Resistant Bacteria will provide advice, information, and recommendations to the Secretary of Health and Human Services regarding the programs and policies developed in the National Action Plan.

Partnerships and Implementation

Implementation of the *National Action Plan* will require the sustained, coordinated, and complementary efforts of individuals and groups around the world, including public and private sector partners, healthcare providers, healthcare leaders, veterinarians, agriculture industry leaders, manufacturers, policymakers, and patients. All of us who depend on antibiotics must join in a common effort to detect, stop, and prevent the emergence and spread of resistant bacteria.

Table 2. Goals and Objectives: Combating Antibiotic-Resistant Bacteria

GOAL 1: Slow the Emergence of Resistant Bacteria and Prevent the Spread of Resistant Infections
Objectives
1.1. Implement public health programs and reporting policies that advance antibiotic-resistance prevention and foster antibiotic stewardship in healthcare settings and the community
1.2. Eliminate the use of medically-important antibiotics for growth promotion in food- producing animals and bring other agricultural uses of antibiotics, for treatment, control, and prevention of disease, under veterinary oversight
1.3. Identify and implement measures to foster stewardship of antibiotics in animals
GOAL 2 : Strengthen National One-Health Surveillance Efforts to Combat Resistance Objectives
2.1. Create a regional public health laboratory network to strengthen national capacity to detect resistant bacterial strains and a specimen repository to facilitate development and evaluation of diagnostic tests and treatments
2.2. Expand and strengthen the national infrastructure for public health surveillance and data reporting, and wprovide incentives for timely reporting of antibiotic-resistance and antibiotic use in all healthcare settings
2.3. Develop, expand, and maintain capacity in State and Federal veterinary and food safety laboratories to conduct antibiotic susceptibility testing and characterize select zoonotic and animal pathogens
2.4. Enhance monitoring of antibiotic-resistance patterns, as well as antibiotic sales, usage, and management practices, at multiple points in the production chain for food animals and retail meat
GOAL 3: Advance Development and Use of Rapid and Innovative Diagnostic Tests for Identification and
Characterization of Resistant Bacteria
Objectives
3.1. Develop and validate new diagnostics—including tests that rapidly distinguish between viral and bacterial pathogens and tests that detect antibiotic-resistance—that can be implemented easily in a wide range of settings
3.2. Expand availability and use of diagnostics to improve treatment of antibiotic-resistant infections, enhance infection control, and facilitate outbreak detection and response in healthcare and community settings
GOAL 4: Accelerate Research to Develop New Antibiotics, Other Therapeutics, Vaccines, and Diagnostics

Objectives
4.1. Conduct research to enhance understanding of environmental factors that facilitate the development of antibiotic-resistance and the spread of resistance genes that are common to animals and humans
4.2. Increase research focused on understanding the nature of microbial communities, how antibiotics affect them, and how they can be harnessed to prevent disease
4.3. Intensify research and development of new therapeutics and vaccines, first-in-class drugs, and new combination therapies for treatment of bacterial infections
4.4. Develop non-traditional therapeutics and innovative strategies to minimize outbreaks caused by resistant bacteria in human and animal populations
4.5. Expand ongoing efforts to provide key data and materials to support the development of promising antibacterial drug candidates
GOAL 5: Improve international collaboration and capacities for prevention, surveillance and antibiotic
research and development
Objectives
Surveillance
5.1. Promote laboratory capability to identify at least 3 of the 7 WHO priority antimicrobial resistant (AMR) pathogens[2] using standardized, reliable detection assays
5.2. Collaborate with WHO, OIE, and other international efforts focused on the development of integrated, laboratory-based surveillance to detect and monitor antibiotic-resistance in relevant animal and human foodborne pathogens
5.3. Develop a mechanism for international communication of critical events that may signify new resistance trends with global public and animal health implications
5.4. Promote the generation and dissemination of information needed to effectively address antibiotic-resistance
Research and Development
5.5. Establish and promote international collaboration and public-private partnerships to incentivize development of new therapeutics to counter antibiotic-resistance including new, next-generation, and other alternatives to antibiotics, vaccines, and affordable, rapidly deployable, point-of-need diagnostics
Prevention and Control
5.6. Support countries to develop and implement national plans to combat antibiotic-resistance and strategies to enhance antimicrobial stewardship
5.7. Partner with other nations to promote quality, safety, and efficacy of antibiotics and strengthen their pharmaceutical supply chains
5.8. Coordinate regulatory approaches by collaborating with international organizations such as FAO and OIE to harmonize international data submission requirements and risk assessment

GOAL 1. SLOW THE EMERGENCE OF RESISTANT BACTERIA AND PREVENT THE SPREAD OF RESISTANT INFECTIONS

Actions taken to achieve Goal 1 will fulfill:

Executive Order 13676, Sections 5 and 7:
– *Improved Antibiotic Stewardship*
– *Preventing and Responding to Infections and Outbreaks with Antibiotic-Resistant Organisms*

Provisions in **PCAST Recommendations #2, #6, and #7:**
– *Effective Surveillance & Response for Antibiotic-resistance*
– *Improving Stewardship of Existing Antibiotics in Health Care*
– *Limit the Use of Antibiotics in Animal Agriculture*

Judicious use of antibiotics in healthcare and agricultural settings is essential to slow the emergence of resistance and extend the useful lifetime of effective antibiotics. Antibiotics are a precious resource, and preserving their usefulness will require cooperation and engagement by healthcare providers, healthcare leaders, pharmaceutical companies, veterinarians, the agricultural industry, and patients. Effective dissemination of information to the public is critical. Prevention of resistance also requires rapid detection and control of infections and outbreaks (see also Goal 2) and regional efforts to control transmission across community and healthcare settings.

Goal 1 includes activities to foster antibiotic stewardship by improving prescribing practices across all healthcare settings, prevent the spread of drug-resistant threats in healthcare facilities and communities, and reduce and eventually eliminate the use of medically-important antibiotics for growth promotion in animals.

By 2020, significant outcomes of Goal 1 will include:

- Establishment of antibiotic stewardship programs in all acute care hospitals and improved antibiotic stewardship across all healthcare settings.
- Reduction of inappropriate antibiotic use by 50% in outpatient settings and by 20% in inpatient settings.

- Establishment of State Antibiotic Resistance (AR) Prevention (Protect) Programs in all 50 states to monitor regionally important multidrug resistant organisms and provide feedback and technical assistance to healthcare facilities.
- Elimination of the use of medically-important antibiotics for growth promotion in food-producing animals.
- Requirement of veterinary oversight for use of medically-important antibiotics in the feed or water of food-producing animals.

1.1. Implement Public Health Programs and Reporting Policies That Advance Antibiotic Resistance Prevention and Foster Antibiotic Stewardship in Healthcare Settings and the Community

Perhaps the single most important action to slow the development and spread of antibiotic-resistant infections is to change the way antibiotics are used. Antibiotics are overprescribed in both human and animal settings, which makes everyone less safe. Investments in this area will be used to develop education and outreach programs to clarify and strengthen responsible, appropriate use of antibiotics in humans and animals. Efforts in this area will help greatly in slowing down the spread of resistant bacteria. This commitment to always use antibiotics appropriately and safely—to use *the right antibiotic at the right time at the right dose for the right duration*—is known as antibiotic stewardship.

Sub-Objective 1.1.1A

Strengthen antibiotic stewardship in inpatient, outpatient, and longterm care settings by expanding existing programs, developing new ones, and monitoring progress and efficacy.

The establishment and expansion of antibiotic stewardship programs will improve patient outcomes and minimize the development of resistance by ensuring judicious use of antibiotics.

Milestones for provision of educational materials to enhance antibiotic stewardship in outpatient settings are provided under Sub-Objective 1.1.1B.

Milestones

Within one year:

- The Departments of Health and Human Services (HHS), Defense (DOD), and Veterans Affairs (VA) will review existing regulations and propose new ones, as needed, requiring hospitals, ambulatory surgery centers, dialysis facilities, and other inpatient facilities to implement robust antibiotic stewardship programs that align with the CDC *Core Elements*. HHS, DOD, and VA will also work together to optimize standardization of stewardship programs and activities, including monitoring activities and reporting criteria.
- The National Healthcare Safety Network (NHSN) will begin tracking the number of healthcare facilities with stewardship policies and programs in place.
- DOD will establish a multidisciplinary group, under the purview of the Assistant Secretary of Defense for Health Affairs, to support and coordinate stewardship activities across DOD.

Within three years:

- All hospitals that participate in Medicare and Medicaid programs must comply with Conditions of Participation (COP). The Centers for Medicare & Medicaid Services (CMS) will issue new COPs or revise current COP *Interpretive Guidelines* to advance compliance with recommendations in CDC's *Core Elements of Hospital Antibiotic Stewardship Programs.* HHS, DOD, and VA will also implement policies that:
    - Encourage implementation of antibiotic stewardship programs as a condition for receiving Federal grants for health care delivery (e.g., in community healthcare centers).
    - Require health facilities operated by the U.S. Government to develop and implement antibiotic stewardship programs and participate in NHSN reporting (see Objective 2.2).
- All acute care hospitals governed by the CMS COP will implement antibiotic stewardship programs. CMS will expand COP requirements to apply to long-term acute care hospitals, other post-acute facilities, ambulatory surgery centers, and dialysis centers.
- CMS will revise existing Interpretive Guidelines (IGs), as needed, to include antimicrobial stewardship improvements. For example, IGs on Quality Assurance and Performance Improvement for hospitals may

incorporate antibiotic-stewardship performance measures developed by the CDC, the Agency for Healthcare Research and Quality (AHRQ), or other professional organizations.

- Training webinars for CMS surveyors will be updated to include information on antibiotic utilization in nursing homes, in accordance with existing IGs in the Infection Control Nursing Home regulations.
- CDC, CMS, AHRQ, and other partners will issue guidance on antibiotic stewardship and best practices for ambulatory surgery centers, dialysis centers, nursing homes and other long-term care facilities, doctors' offices and other outpatient settings, pharmacies, emergency departments, and medical departments at correctional facilities.
- At least 25 States, the District of Columbia, and Puerto Rico will establish or enhance antibiotic stewardship activities in inpatient healthcare delivery settings, in accordance with the CDC *Core Elements*. CDC will support these efforts via State AR Prevention (Protect) Programs for Healthcare ("AR Protect Programs"; see also Sub-Objective 1.1.2).

Within five years:

- DOD will support antibiotic stewardship programs and interventions critical for maintaining quality health care throughout the Military Healthcare System (MHS).
- CDC will work with select hospital systems to expand antibiotic use reporting and stewardship implementation, and will partner with nursing organizations to develop and implement stewardship programs and interventions in a set of nursing homes.
- All states will establish or enhance antibiotic stewardship activities in healthcare delivery settings.

Sub-Objective 1.1.1B

Strengthen educational programs that inform physicians, veterinarians, members of the agricultural industry, and the public about good antibiotic stewardship.

Educational programs that promote good antibiotic stewardship in healthcare settings include:

- *Get Smart: Know When Antibiotics Work.* Many antibiotics prescribed in doctors' offices, clinics, and other outpatient settings are not needed. This program focuses on appropriate antibiotic prescribing and use for common illnesses in children and adults.

- *Get Smart for Healthcare.* Many patients in hospitals, nursing homes, and other healthcare facilities receive antibiotics to fight infections, but these drugs are often prescribed incorrectly. This program helps clinicians prescribe *the right drugs for the right patients at the right doses and times.*

The United States Department of Agriculture (USDA), CDC, and the Food and Drug Administration (FDA) will also continue to work with partners in the agriculture industry to advance appropriate use of antibiotics in food animals and promote collaborations among partners in medicine, veterinary medicine, and public health.

Additional milestones for provision of educational materials to enhance antibiotic stewardship in agricultural settings are provided under Sub-Objectives 1.2.3 and 1.3.1.

Milestones

Within one year:

- CDC and VA will apply lessons learned from the CDC and VA pilot project to provide clinicians with support for making prescribing decisions based on judicious use of antibiotics and will submit a manuscript for publication describing initial research findings from this effort.

Within three years:

- CDC will support public health departments in establishing statewide programs for antibiotic stewardship and appropriate antibiotic use. These programs will identify healthcare facilities with high antibiotic-prescribing rates and use lessons learned from the CDC and VA pilot project (see above) and other best practices to improve antibiotic prescribing in these facilities. The success of these efforts will be assessed by measuring changes in prescribing rates and in clinicians' understanding of antibiotic stewardship activities and programs.
- CDC will provide technical assistance to Federal facilities (e.g., those operated by DOD, the VA, and the Indian Health Service) and other large health systems in scaling up implementation and assessment of interventions to improve outpatient antibiotic prescribing, extending

effective interventions to long-term care settings, and ensuring long-term sustainability of antibiotic stewardship efforts.

- DOD will initiate the planning and approval process to modify clinical decision-support interventions in DOD facilities in targeted regions.
- CDC, CMS, and partners will propose expanded quality measures for antibiotic prescribing.
- CMS will expand the Physician Quality Reporting System (PQRS) to include quality measures that discourage inappropriate antibiotic use to treat non-bacterial infections, such as respiratory tract infections.
- CDC will expand training and support to acute care facilities and nursing homes to improve antibiotic stewardship, as part of the *Get Smart for Healthcare* project.

Within five years:

- CDC will evaluate the impact of quality measures on antibiotic use and provide feedback to healthcare partners.

Additionally, CDC will continue to host a *Get Smart About Antibiotics Week* observance each November to raise public awareness about antibiotic-resistance and the importance of appropriate antibiotic prescribing.

Sub-Objective 1.1.2

Expand collaborative efforts by groups of healthcare facilities that focus on preventing the spread of antibiotic-resistant bacteria that pose a serious threat to public health (Table 3).

Public health action to prevent transmission of healthcare-associated infections—including drug-resistant bacterial infections—has traditionally been taken by individual healthcare facilities. However, drug-resistant organisms—including multidrug resistant organisms (MDROs) such as CRE and MRSA, and *Clostridium difficile* infections that are associated with antibiotic use (Table 3)—can spread regionally from one healthcare facility to another when patients colonized or infected with resistant bacteria move between hospitals or long-term care facilities within a state or locality. It is therefore imperative that healthcare facilities work together, in close partnership with state health departments, to implement effective interventions that slow the regional spread of drug-resistant pathogens.

Milestones

Within one year:

- The DOD Multidrug-Resistant Organism Repository & Surveillance Network (MRSN) will expand its detection and reporting capabilities to include *Clostridium difficile* and other high-risk drug-resistant pathogens.

Within three years:

- At least 25 states, the District of Columbia, and Puerto Rico will establish or enhance State AR Prevention (Protect) Programs to improve antibiotic use and reduce transmission of resistant pathogens. Activities will include measuring the incidence of at least one regionally important MDRO, providing healthcare facilities with feedback on local and regional MDRO rates, and providing healthcare facilities with technical assistance to advance MDRO prevention. CDC and CMS Quality Improvement Networks (QINs) will work with state and large local health departments to advance these efforts. QINs are groups of health quality experts, clinicians, and consumers who help improve the care delivered to people with Medicare.
- At least 20 state health departments will maintain advanced capacity for rapid response to drug-resistant gonorrhea, including capacity to detect, diagnose, and investigate suspected resistant cases within their state or region and assist healthcare providers in providing appropriate treatment of infected patients.

Within five years:

- CDC will expand capacity to prevent the importation of cases of multidrug resistant Tuberculosis (TB) (MDR-TB) by doubling TB screening among migrants from high-incidence countries from 500,000 to 1 million persons per year.
- State AR Prevention (Protect) Programs will be in place in all 50 states, as well as the District of Columbia and Puerto Rico.

Sub-Objective 1.1.3

Implement annual reporting of antibiotic use in inpatient and outpatient settings and identify geographic variations and/or variations at the provider and/ or patient level that can help guide interventions.

Antibiotic resistance in healthcare settings is a significant threat to public health. Because nearly all Americans receive care in a healthcare setting at some point in their lives, the problem can affect anyone. Patients undergoing chemotherapy for cancer and very sick patients in intensive care units are at special risk, because they are already vulnerable due to weakened immune systems and underlying illness.

Through its antibiotic use (AU) and antimicrobial resistance (AR) modules, the National Health Safety Network (NHSN) receives hospital data on:

- Amounts of specific antibiotics used to treat hospitalized patients (AU reporting).
- Cases of drug-resistant disease (AR reporting).

The AU and AR data allow healthcare facilities to target areas of concern, make needed improvements, and track the success of their efforts. NHSN data also allow CDC to track regional and national trends in drug resistant diseases and provide hospitals with feedback about prescribing practices and antibiotic stewardship.

Milestones for AU reporting are provided below, as part of the effort to foster antibiotic stewardship. Additional milestones for AR reporting and for strengthening the public health surveillance infrastructure that supports AU and AR reporting are provided in Goal 2.

Milestones: Reporting Antibiotic Use in Inpatient Settings

Within one year:

- CDC will finalize arrangements for the purchase of proprietary data on inpatient antibiotic use to supplement NHSN data until a larger number of hospitals begin to utilize the NHSN module for antibiotic use reporting.
- CDC will work with healthcare and public health partners to propose new healthcare-facility antibiotic use measures to the National Quality Forum (NQF; see also Sub-Objective 2.2.1).

Within three years:

- CDC will use data collected through the NHSN AU module to provide annual national estimates of aggregated inpatient antibiotic use and feedback to healthcare facilities on antibiotic use, indicating whether antibiotic use rates are above or below the national average.

- CDC will establish routine reporting of antibiotic use and resistance data from select hospital systems via the NHSN AU and AR modules (see Objective 2.2).
- DOD will centralize its reporting of inpatient antibiotic use to NHSN.

Within five years:

- CDC will provide estimates of inappropriate inpatient antibiotic prescribing rates by state and region and use this data to target and prioritize intervention efforts.

Milestones: Reporting Antibiotic Use in Outpatient Settings

Within one year:

- CDC will report outpatient prescribing rates for 2011 and 2012 and use this data to target and prioritize intervention efforts.
- CDC will establish a benchmark (in terms of prescriptions per population) for reduction in antibiotic use.

Within three years:

- Starting in 2016, CDC will issue yearly reports on progress in meeting the national target of 50% reduction in inappropriate use of antibiotics in outpatient settings (see above), as well as on overall trends in antibiotic prescribing.
- DOD will establish goals for reducing antibiotic use in DOD facilities that provide outpatient care for military personnel and their families.
- DOD will centralize reporting of outpatient antibiotic use and issue annual summary reports.

Sub-Objective 1.1.4

Develop and pilot new interventions to address geographic, sociocultural, policy, economic, and clinical drivers of the emergence and spread of antibiotic-resistance and misuse or overuse of antibiotics.

Milestones

Within one year:

- The Agency for Healthcare Research and Quality (AHRQ) and CDC will host a meeting of experts and stakeholders to consider knowledge gaps for prevention of antibiotic-resistant, healthcare-associated infections and identify potential interventions for development, field testing, and eventual widespread implementation.
- CDC Emerging Infections Program (EIP) sites will perform assessments of antibiotic use and resistance to allow updating of national estimates of antibiotic-resistant, healthcare-associated infections and of antibiotic-resistance threats in the United States.
- CDC EIP sites will solicit applications for funding large-scale interventions to reduce *C. difficile* infections through enhanced antibiotic stewardship programs.

Within three years:

- The CDC Prevention Epicenters Program will evaluate one or more novel antibiotic-resistance prevention tools for use in diverse healthcare settings.
- CDC EIP sites will initiate large-scale demonstration projects to field-test AR interventions developed by the Prevention Epicenters Program.
- AHRQ will sponsor research to develop improved methods and approaches for combating antibiotic-resistance and conducting antibiotic stewardship activities in multiple healthcare settings, with a focus on long-term and ambulatory care centers, as well as acute care hospitals. AHRQ will support translation of research findings into antibiotic-resistance prevention tools that can be implemented by healthcare providers in long-term and ambulatory care settings, as well as in hospitals.
- CDC will perform two randomized control trials to test improved treatment methods to prevent the spread of MDR-TB.

Within five years:

- CDC will finalize data collection to validate new antibiotic-resistance prevention tools tested by the EIP sites and transition validated interventions to ongoing State AR Prevention (Protect) Programs.

Sub-Objective 1.1.5

Streamline regulatory processes for updating and approving or clearing antibiotic susceptibility testing devices, as appropriate, so that clinicians receive up-to-date interpretive criteria to guide antibacterial drug selection.

Manufacturers of antibiotic susceptibility testing (AST) devices provide interpretive criteria that are used by healthcare providers to categorize a bacterial isolate as "susceptible" or "resistant" to particular antibiotics. However, when bacteria develop new means of resistance, the interpretive criteria may no longer be clinically useful. Rapid updating of interpretive criteria in AST devices—by manufacturers or by standards development organizations (SDOs)—is therefore essential to provide accurate information to guide appropriate drug treatment.

Milestones

Within one year:

- FDA will provide technical assistance, as appropriate, on legislative proposals being considered to streamline updating of interpretive criteria for AST devices.

Within five years:

- FDA will update AST interpretive criteria more efficiently and rapidly (e.g., by adopting criteria developed by SDOs rather than including interpretive guidelines on labels).

1.2. Eliminate the Use of Medically Important Antibiotics for Growth Promotion in Food-Producing Animals and Bring under Veterinary Oversight Other in-Feed and in-Water Uses of Antibiotics That Are Medically Important for Treatment, Control, and Prevention of Disease

FDA's strategy to ensure the judicious use of medically important antibiotics in animal agriculture is outlined in two guidance documents:

- FDA Guidance for Industry (GFI) #209—*The Judicious Use of Medically Important Antimicrobial Drugs in Food-Producing Animals*—is intended to limit medically important antimicrobial drugs to uses in animals that (1) are considered necessary for assuring animal health, and (2) include veterinary oversight or consultation.

- FDA Guidance for Industry (GFI) #213—*New Animal Drugs and New Animal Drug Combination Products Administered in or on Medicated Feed or Drinking Water of Food-Producing Animals: Recommendations for Drug Sponsors for Voluntarily Aligning Product Use Conditions with GFI #209*—calls for:
  - Voluntary revision of the FDA-approved use conditions on the labels of medically important antibiotics to remove production indications, such as increased rate of weight gain and improved feed efficiency.
  - Phasing in veterinary oversight of the remaining therapeutic uses of medically important antibiotics in feed or water by changing the current over-the-counter status of these drugs. Because antibiotics in feed or water are typically administered to herds or flocks of food-producing animals, in-feed or in-water antibiotic use leads to an increased risk of selecting for resistance.

Sub-Objective 1.2.1

Implement FDA GFI #213 to eliminate the use of medically important antibiotics for growth promotion in animals and bring other in-feed and in-water uses of medically important antibiotics under veterinary oversight. FDA should evaluate the adoption of the proposed changes under GFI #213 after the three-year implementation period and take further action as appropriate.

Milestones

Within one year:

- FDA will finalize changes to the Veterinary Feed Directive (VFD) regulation to encourage manufacturers to transition the dispensing status of in-feed antibiotics covered by GFI #213 from over-the-counter (OTC) to VFD status, which requires veterinary oversight. FDA will publish an enhanced summary report of antibiotics sold or distributed for use in food-producing animals from 2009 to 2013. This report will support the effort to monitor the antibiotic usage aspects of Guidance #213 (see also Objective 2.2.4).

Within three years:

- FDA, in partnership with animal drug sponsors, will complete all changes recommended by GFI #213 and GFI #209. Once these changes are complete, growth promotion uses of medically important antibiotics will no longer be permitted, and the use of medically important antibiotics in the feed or water of food-producing animals will require veterinary oversight.

Sub-Objective 1.2.2

Assess progress toward eliminating the use of medically important antibiotics for growth promotion in food-producing animals through enhanced data collection on antibiotic sales and use.

Milestones

Within five years:

- FDA, in partnership with USDA and the animal agricultural industry, will evaluate and report on the impact of GFI #213 by analyzing data on antibiotic use, including total sales of antibiotics in animal agriculture and types and prevalence of antibiotic-resistance among selected foodborne pathogens and commensals isolated from retail meat and farm animals.

Milestones for enhancing collection of data to monitor the impact of GFI #213 in fostering the judicious use of antibiotics in food-producing animals are provided under Objective 2.4.

Sub-Objective 1.2.3

Develop and implement educational outreach efforts to ensure that veterinarians and animal producers receive information and training to support implementation of these changes.

Within three years:

- FDA will collaborate with veterinary organizations, animal producer organizations, the animal feed industry, and others to develop and implement educational outreach efforts to ensure that veterinarians and animal producers receive the necessary information and training to support implementation of GFI #213 (see also: Sub-Objective 1.3.1).

Sub-Objective 1.2.4

Optimize public awareness about progress toward eliminating the use of medically important antibiotics for animal-growth promotion.

Within one year:

- FDA will publish and maintain a public web listing of products affected by GFI #213.
- FDA will begin publishing periodic updates summarizing progress in adoption of the changes proposed in GFI #213.

Within three years:

- FDA will publish a final assessment of the progress of GFI #213 on eliminating the use of medically important antibiotics for animal-growth promotion.

1.3. Identify and Implement Measures to Foster Stewardship of Antibiotics in Animals

Sub-Objective 1.3.1

Develop, implement, and measure the effectiveness of evidence-based educational outreach to veterinarians and animal producers to advance antibiotic stewardship and judicious use of antibiotics in agricultural settings.

Milestones

Within one year:

- FDA and USDA will consult with livestock and veterinary organizations on the development of educational outreach materials on judicious use of antibiotics and antibiotic stewardship, and will meet with the American Veterinary Medical Association and the American Association of Veterinary Medical Colleges to consider the incorporation of additional material on antibiotic resistance and antibiotic stewardship into the curricula of U.S. veterinary colleges.
- USDA will conduct assessments in various animal production and veterinary settings to identify priority areas in which research is needed to support the development and validation of stewardship activities to assure judicious antibiotic use.

- USDA will solicit applications to the USDA Antimicrobial Resistance Initiative Program, which aims to advance development and use of antibiotic stewardship practices that assure judicious use of antibiotics in agriculture. Applicants may propose a combination of activities, including research studies and development of educational and outreach materials. Projected outcomes of the educational and outreach activities include better preparation of the next generation of veterinarians and laboratory scientists. Projected outcomes of the research activities include development of sustainable strategies to mitigate antibiotic resistance (see Objective 4).

Within 3 years:

- USDA will support the distribution of educational and outreach materials on antibiotic stewardship and judicious use of antibiotics that target veterinarians, producers, educators, and consumers. These activities will be accomplished through the Antimicrobial Resistance Initiative awardees whose integrated projects are linked to the Cooperative Extension System for education and extension/outreach activities.

Sub-Objective 1.3.2

Foster collaborations and public-private partnerships with public health, pharmaceutical, and agricultural stakeholders to facilitate identification and implementation of interventions (e.g., good husbandry practices) to reduce the spread of antibiotic-resistance.

Milestones

Within one year:

- FDA and USDA will identify priority areas for research to develop and validate stewardship activities to reduce the spread of antibiotic-resistance.
- FDA and USDA will work with livestock and veterinary organizations to consider ways to develop, update, and incorporate assessments of antibiotic stewardship activities into quality assurance programs.

Within three years:

- FDA and USDA will support applied research in field settings to demonstrate the feasibility and effectiveness of stewardship programs and test and validate alternatives to traditional uses of antibiotics in agriculture.

Within five years:

- FDA and USDA will identify validated interventions to reduce the spread of antibiotic resistance and work with public and private sector partners to incorporate them into veterinary practice.

Sub-Objective 1.3.3

Identify, develop, and revise key agricultural practices that allow timely and effective implementation of interventions that improve animal health and efficient production.

Milestones

Within three years:

- FDA and USDA will support drivers-of-change studies to determine which stewardship materials and educational approaches are most effective in improving antibiotic use practices.

Sub-Objective 1.3.4

Develop appropriate metrics to gauge the success of stewardship efforts and guide their continued evolution and optimization.

Milestones

Within three years:

- FDA and USDA will:
    - Collect additional data regarding antibiotic use and resistance in food-producing animals. These data will supplement existing surveillance data used to evaluate the impact of GFI #213 on use practices and resistance trends over time.
    - Measure changes in antibiotic stewardship programs and practices as part of quality assurance programs in cattle operations and swine and broiler chicken production.

- Use baseline data from the National Animal Health Monitoring System (NAHMS), where available, to evaluate changes over a 5-year time horizon.

GOAL 2. STRENGTHEN NATIONAL ONE-HEALTH SURVEILLANCE EFFORTS TO COMBAT RESISTANCE

Actions taken to achieve Goal 2 will fulfill:

Executive Order 13676, Section 6:
– *Strengthening National Surveillance Efforts for Resistant Bacteria*
Provisions in **PCAST Recommendations #2 and #6:**
– *Effective Surveillance & Response for Antibiotic Resistance*
– *Improving Stewardship of Existing Antibiotics in Health Care*

The “One-Health” approach to disease surveillance for human and animal pathogens is critical to combat antibiotic-resistance. Improved detection and control can be achieved through enhancement and integration of data from surveillance systems that monitor human pathogens and commensals—including NHSN, the Emerging Infections Program (EIP), and the National Antimicrobial Resistance Monitoring System (NARMS)—with data from surveillance systems that monitor animal pathogens—including the National Animal Health Monitoring System (NAHMS), the National Animal Health Laboratory Network (NAHLN), and the Veterinary Laboratory Investigation and Response Network (Vet-LIRN). These activities will provide high-quality data, including detailed genomic data, and other information necessary to track resistant bacteria in diverse settings in a timely fashion.

Goal 2 activities include creation of a Detect Network of Antimicrobial Resistance (AR) Regional Laboratories that will provide a standardized platform for resistance testing and advanced capacity for genetic characterization of resistant bacteria, including whole genome sequencing. In addition, Goal 2 activities will enhance monitoring of antibiotic sales, usage, resistance and management practices at multiple points along in the food-production chain, from farms to processing plants to supermarkets.

By 2020, significant outcomes of Goal 2 will include:

- Creation of a regional public health network—the Detect Network of AR Regional Laboratories— for resistance testing, a specimen repository for resistant bacterial strains, and a National Sequence Database of Resistant Pathogens.
- Routine reporting of antibiotic use and resistance data to NHSN by 95% of Medicare-eligible hospitals, as well as by DOD and VA healthcare facilities.
- Routine testing of zoonotic and animal pathogens for antibiotic susceptibility at ten to twenty NAHLN and Vet-LIRN member laboratories, using standardized testing methods and data-sharing practices.
- Publication of enhanced summary reports on the sale and distribution of antibiotics approved for use in food-producing animals, issued on an annual basis.

2.1. Create a Regional Public Health Laboratory Network to Strengthen National Capacity to Detect Resistant Bacterial Strains, and Create a Specimen Repository to Facilitate Development and Evaluation of Diagnostic Tests and Treatments

Sub-Objective 2.1.1

Create a regional public health laboratory network that uses standardized testing platforms to expand the availability of reference testing services, characterize emerging resistance patterns and bacterial strains obtained from outbreaks and other sources, and facilitate rapid data analysis and dissemination of information.

Milestones

Within one year:

- CDC will develop an implementation plan for the Detect Network of AR Regional Laboratories that considers all aspects of operation, including specimen transport, testing, reporting, and data-sharing.

- Multidrug-resistant Organism Repository & Surveillance Network (MRSN) will be formally recognized as a reference laboratory network with responsibility for reporting data on antibiotic resistance and antibiotic use in military treatment facilities. It will expand its mission to include rapid characterization of emerging resistance patterns, laboratory support during outbreak investigations, and reporting of clinically relevant bacterial pathogens for facilities that serve military service members and their families.

Within three years:

- CDC will designate at least five public health laboratories as part of the Detect Network of Regional AR Laboratories, which is charged with rapid detection of outbreaks caused by drug-resistant pathogens, characterization of resistance mechanisms, and tracking resistance trends and identifying emerging forms of resistance. CDC will work with DOD and USDA to share resistance detection strategies and protocols.
- CDC will work with the Association of Public Health Laboratories (APHL), state and local health laboratories, and other partners to provide technical assistance and guidance to the Regional AR Laboratories, as needed.

Sub-Objective 2.1.2

Link data generated by the regional public health laboratory network to existing public health surveillance networks so that antibiotic susceptibility testing data are immediately available to local, state, and Federal public health authorities as they detect and investigate outbreaks, as well as to veterinary diagnostic and food safety laboratory databases and/or surveillance systems, as needed.

Milestones

Within three years:

- The five designated Detect Network Regional AR Laboratories (Sub-Objective 2.1.1) will be integrated into an AR communications network that posts early warning alerts and reports urgent results and trends.
- The AR communication network will establish linkages with DOD and VA clinical, veterinary, and food safety laboratories.

Sub-Objective 2.1.3

Create a repository of resistant bacterial strains (an "isolate bank") and maintain a well-curated reference database that describes the characteristics of these strains. The repository will aid biotechnology and pharmaceutical companies that develop new antibiotics and therapeutics and/or design next-generation tests, diagnostic test developers and regulatory agencies who evaluate these tests, government facilities, academic labs, and pharmaceutical companies that test antibiotics for clinical effectiveness and researchers, regulators, and others who assess the effectiveness of interventions to prevent resistance.

Milestones

Within one year:

- CDC and FDA will develop a defined set of microorganisms to be included in a repository of resistant bacterial strains, including the urgent and serious threats listed in Table 1, and a bioinformatics database to maintain detailed information on the drug susceptibilities and resistance mechanisms of each repository strain.
- The DOD will post data on a representative sample of characterized isolates on a website that can be accessed by authenticated users.

Within three years:

- CDC and FDA will create the repository and database for resistant bacterial strains and, in conjunction with DOD, will provide isolates to diagnostic test manufacturers and research laboratories, as needed.
- DOD will continue to maintain its repository of resistant bacterial strains within the MRSN, update procedures for specimen collection, storage, and data-sharing, and share information, as appropriate, with industry, academic, non-profit, and government stakeholders.

Annually thereafter:

- CDC and FDA will update the repository of bacterial strains, incorporating isolates with new resistance mechanisms or emerging resistance patterns identified by the national infectious disease surveillance system.
- CDC, FDA, and DOD will update procedures for strain collection, storage, and data-sharing.

Sub-Objective 2.1.4

Develop and maintain a national sequence database of resistant pathogens.

Milestones

Within one year:

- FDA and the National Institutes of Health (NIH) will pilot-test a sequence database containing more than 550 drug-resistant bacterial strains, with accompanying clinical and demographic data ("metadata"). The entries will cover a range of organisms selected by CDC to assist in diagnostic development.
- NIH and partners will sequence additional high-priority, drug-resistant strains to add to the database.
- DOD will stand up its diagnostic sequence database, inclusive of genomic information (including raw reads and interpretations /annotations) and relevant phenotypic metadata for access by authenticated users.

Within three years:

- FDA and NIH will review the pilot project to address challenges and identify lessons learned concerning data standards, analysis tools, and data-sharing (see also Objective 4.2).
- As new strains are added to the repository of resistant strains described in Sub-Objective 2.1.3, NIH, FDA, and CDC will work with public and private sector partners to add the genomic sequences of each isolate to the database.
- NIH will expand the pilot project database into a National Database of Resistant Pathogens (NDRP) that will continue to incorporate information on newly identified bacterial strains. The database entries will be cross-referenced with entries in the bioinformatics database described in Sub-Objective 2.1.3.

2.2. Expand and Strengthen the National Infrastructure for Public Health Surveillance and Data Reporting, and Provide Incentives for Timely Reporting of Antibiotic-Resistance and Antibiotic Use in All Healthcare Settings

The milestones below cover improvements in reporting infrastructure that pertain to both antibiotic resistance (AR) reporting and antibiotic use (AU) reporting. Additional milestones for AU reporting are provided under Objective 1.1.3 as part of the effort to advance antibiotic stewardship in healthcare facilities.

Sub-Objective 2.2.1

Enhance reporting infrastructure and provide incentives for reporting (e.g., require reporting of antibiotic-resistance data to NHSN as part of the CMS Hospital Inpatient Quality Reporting Program).

Within one year:

- CDC will submit proposals for new measures for hospital reporting of data on antibiotic use to the National Quality Forum (NQF).
- CDC will create a user-friendly electronic portal that makes aggregated NHSN data publicly available and facilitates integrated analyses of state and regional trends and practices.

Within three years:

- CDC will submit proposals for new measures for hospital reporting of data on antibiotic resistance to NQF.
- CDC will work with CMS and public health partners to minimize the regulatory burden and maximize the health utility of requiring hospitals to report antibiotic use and resistance to NHSN as part of the CMS Hospital Inpatient Quality Reporting (IQR) Program. Data will be reported through the NHSN AU and AR modules.
- Once the analysis has been completed and new NQF measures have been approved, CMS will begin the process of proposing new IQR rules.
- CDC will work with DOD and VA to define steps and resource needs to support NHSN data submission by DOD and VHA facilities and ensure timely analysis of trends in antibiotic use and antibiotic resistance.
- CDC will expand user-support and validation programs to accommodate expected increases in hospital reporting through the NHSN AU and AR modules during 2017-2019.

Within five years:

- CDC will work with hospital consortiums and state-based hospital networks to determine whether additional reporting incentives are needed in place of (or in addition to) reporting required by CMS.

Sub-Objective 2.2.2

Add electronic reporting of antibiotic use and resistance data in a standard file format to the Stage 3 Meaningful Use certification program for electronic health record systems.

To qualify for an incentive payment through the CMS Medicare Electronic Health Records (EHR) Incentive Program, eligible hospitals must adopt certified EHR technology and use it to achieve specific objectives. The objectives for Stage 1 were *data capture and data sharing.* The objective for Stage 2 was *advance clinical processes.* The objective for Stage 3, *improved outcomes,* can be achieved by using EHR to report antibiotic use and resistance data to CDC via the NHSN AU and AR modules.

Milestones

Within one year:

- CDC will provide technical assistance to hospitals across the nation that report drug-resistance data to NHSN via the NHSN AU and AR modules.

Within three years:

- CMS will finalize a tool to help software developers certify electronic health records and other health IT software, as appropriate, for recording and submitting AU data.
- CMS will complete an analysis of standards and terminologies for AU reporting to ensure alignment between NHSN reporting and IQR reporting and to support local clinical decision-making.

Within five years:

- CDC and partners will develop an AU electronic clinical-quality NHSN-reporting measure in a standard file format that hospitals can use to achieve the Stage 3 Meaningful Use objective and accelerate reporting. The timing of this activity will depend on the timeframe of the CMS Meaningful Use certification program.
- Once an AU electronic clinical-quality NHSN-reporting measure has been developed, it will be submitted to NQF for review and endorsement and to CMS for consideration as a reporting requirement of the CMS Hospital Inpatient Quality Reporting Program.

Sub-Objective 2.2.3

Expand the activities and scope of the Emerging Infections Program (EIP) to include monitoring of additional urgent and serious bacterial threats (see Table 3) and evaluating populations at risk across community and healthcare settings.

The EIP, a network of 10 state health departments,[3] conducts active, population-based surveillance for infectious diseases of public health importance. AR surveillance is conducted for ten of the 15 urgent and serious threats listed in Table 1:

- *Clostridium difficile* (10 sites)
- Carbapenem-resistant *Enterobacteriaceae* (CRE; 8 sites)
- Multidrug-resistant *Acinetobacter* (8 sites)
- Drug-resistant *Candida* (4 sites)
- Methicillin-resistant *Staphylococcus aureus* (MRSA; 9 sites)
- Drug-resistant *Streptococcus pneumoniae* (10 sites)
- Drug-resistant foodborne pathogens, including *Campylobacter, Shigella*, *Salmonella Typhi*, and non-typhoidal *Salmonella* (10 sites)

Milestones

Within one year:

- CDC will host a meeting of EIP Principal Investigators to consider ways to improve EIP surveillance for drug-resistant threats. The outcomes of this meeting will include refined protocols and standard operating procedures to enable EIP surveillance of additional threats in additional EIP sites.
- CDC EIP sites will pilot methodology to incorporate at least one additional urgent or serious threat into surveillance activities.

Within three years:

- CDC will establish up to 10 additional EIP sites, including sites in the West and Midwest that will monitor drug-resistant pathogens. CDC will evaluate the contribution of these new sites to collection of data that better represents the incidence and prevalence of drug-resistant disease in the United States.
- CDC EIP sites will initiate a study to evaluate populations at risk for CRE.

- CDC will work with research partners and EIP sites to validate molecular assays to support surveillance for drug-resistant gonorrhea.

Within five years:

- CDC will expand EIP activities to include surveillance for additional urgent and serious AR threats (Table 3).
- EIP will help coordinate a public health surveillance study to explore the impact of bacterial populations within the human microbiome on attack rates of drug-resistant pathogens (e.g., *C. difficile*, CRE, MRSA, *Candida, Salmonella, Shigella, Campylobacter,* and *S. pneumoniae*).
- CDC will analyze the resistance of bacteria in the intestines of healthy people with a variety of diets, lifestyles, and antibiotic-use histories.

Over the following years:

- The EIP network will continue to conduct active surveillance for drug-resistant bacteria, provide data to inform CDC's AR threat reports, identify populations at special risk, and test interventions to reduce the emergence and spread of AR threats.

2.3. Develop, Expand, and Maintain Capacity in Veterinary and Food Safety Laboratories to Conduct Standardized Antibiotic Susceptibility Testing and Characterize Select Zoonotic and Animal Pathogens

Surveillance for antibiotic-resistant zoonotic and animal pathogens may be enhanced nationwide by building capacity among member laboratories of the USDA National Animal Health Laboratory Network (NAHLN), the FDA Veterinary Laboratory Investigation and Response Network (Vet-LIRN), and USDA-Food Safety and Inspection Service (FSIS) Field Service Laboratories. NAHLN is managed by the National Veterinary Services Laboratories (NVSL).

Sub-Objective 2.3.1

Expand and maintain veterinary and food safety laboratory infrastructure for the identification of select zoonotic and animal health pathogens through the implementation of new diagnostic technologies (see also Goal 3).

Milestones

Within one year:

- USDA and FDA will assess current capacities and protocols within NAHLN and Vet-LIRN member laboratories and identify capacity development needs to support nationwide AR surveillance for zoonotic pathogens and pathogens of importance to animal health.

Within three years:

- USDA and FDA will support capacity development in ten selected NAHLN and Vet-LIRN member laboratories by providing training in standardized methodologies for antibiotic-susceptibility testing.
- USDA and FDA will provide support to five or more NAHLN and/or Vet-LIRN member laboratories for next-generation sequencing equipment and training on the use of whole-genome sequencing techniques and bioinformatics.

Within five years:

- Ten to twenty NAHLN and Vet-LIRN member laboratories will establish capacity and infrastructure for antibiotic susceptibility testing of bacterial isolates using standardized testing methods (involving WGS or other techniques) and data-sharing mechanisms.

Sub-Objective 2.3.2

Accelerate and standardize antibiotic susceptibility testing and bacterial characterization for select zoonotic and animal health pathogens, coordinating with appropriate stakeholder groups.

Milestones

Within one year:

- USDA and FDA will develop standardized protocols for assessing proficiency in susceptibility testing.

Within three years:

- USDA and FDA will launch pilot projects in three to five NAHLN and/or Vet-LIRN laboratories to establish proficiency in conducting standardized antibiotic susceptibility testing.

Within five years:

- Ten to twenty NAHLN and/or Vet-LIRN member laboratories will actively conduct antibiotic susceptibility testing using standardized methodologies.

Sub-Objective 2.3.3

Enhance communications and identify mechanisms for sharing and reporting antibiotic-susceptibility data on select zoonotic and animal health pathogens collected by veterinary diagnostic and food safety laboratories. These data should be stored in a centralized repository that can be linked with relevant public health databases, as appropriate, while maintaining source confidentiality.

Milestones

Within one year:

- USDA and FDA will initiate discussions with veterinary diagnostic and food safety laboratories to identify opportunities and incentives to share antibiotic-susceptibility data and consider barriers such as confidentiality concerns that would prevent or incentives that would encourage this type of data sharing among NAHLN and Vet-LIRN laboratories.

Within three years:

- USDA and FDA will identify requirements for a system to facilitate national collection, analysis, and reporting of antibiotic-susceptibility testing data by NAHLN and/or Vet-LIRN laboratories, develop guidelines for data collection and for sharing metadata, and generate mechanisms and criteria for linking veterinary data to public health data (e.g., by entering veterinary data into the NARMS database).
- USDA and FDA will launch pilot projects in three to five NAHLN and/or Vet-LIRN laboratories for data collection and sharing.

Within five years:

- USDA and FDA will establish an IT system that links NAHLN and Vet-LIRN laboratories that conduct antibiotic susceptibility testing and facilitates sharing, analysis, and reporting of veterinary AR data through a centralized repository.

2.4. Enhance Monitoring of Antibiotic-Resistance Patterns, As Well As Antibiotic Sales, Usage, and Management Practices, at Multiple Points in the Production Chain for Food Animals and Retail Meat

Additional baseline information regarding on-farm use of antibiotics is urgently needed to:

- Monitor the impact of FDA Guidance for Industry #213 in fostering the judicious use of antibiotics in food-producing animals (see Goal 1.2).
- Investigate whether certain antibiotic use practices in food production facilitate the development of resistance.

Currently, NAHMS collects voluntary information on on-farm use and resistance patterns on a periodic basis. However, there is increased need for on-farm antibiotic-use data, and the relationship between use and resistance requires enhanced data collection. As yet, no system is in place to provide detailed surveillance data on the use of antibiotics in agriculture or associations between antibiotic use and the development of resistance.

Sub-Objective 2.4.1

Enhance surveillance of antibiotic resistance in animal and zoonotic pathogens and commensal organisms by strengthening the National Antimicrobial Resistance Monitoring System (NARMS) and leveraging other field- and laboratory-based surveillance systems.

Milestones

Within one year:

- USDA will develop a plan to enhance efforts to monitor the occurrence of drug-resistant zoonotic pathogens in food animals on farms and at slaughter.

Within three years:

- CDC will decrease by 50% the time required to detect and characterize drug-resistant enteric pathogens through NARMS surveillance, and communicate results to stakeholders.

- CDC will improve the detection, investigation, and mitigation of multistate outbreaks caused by resistant enteric bacteria through a 25% reduction in time from the initial notification to NARMS to reporting of susceptibility testing results.
- CDC will gather risk factor information, including data on recent antibiotic use, foreign travel, medical conditions, non-food exposures, and health outcomes for patients with drug-resistant infections. This data (including information about sources of infection) will be used to help improve antibiotic prescribing practices, reduce invasive infections, and decrease hospitalization rates.
- CDC will identify resistance patterns for Salmonella by analyzing near-real-time data from all Salmonella isolates sent to public health laboratories. This activity will help detect outbreaks earlier and faster, improve health outcomes, and avert large food recalls.
- CDC will conduct susceptibility testing on an increased proportion of Campylobacter isolates to help identify outbreaks and determine the sources of drug-resistant Campylobacter infections.
- USDA will implement routine susceptibility testing of veterinary diagnostic isolates and report its findings.
- USDA-FSIS will expand its meat sample and cecal sample[42] surveillance for antibiotic resistance, in collaboration with FDA, NARMS, and other USDA offices.
- FDA will expand retail meat sampling to improve the representativeness of surveillance data on bacterial contamination of meat products.

Within five years:

- NARMS will partner with NHSN to obtain drug-resistance data from clinical laboratories on bacteria isolated from persons with invasive *Salmonella*, *Campylobacter*, or *Shigella* infections. Analysis of this data will provide much-needed information about the burdens and outcomes of drug-resistant enteric infections.
- CDC will begin a pilot project to evaluate the association between antibiotic-resistant urinary tract infections and foodborne bacteria.

Sub-Objective 2.4.2

Enhance collection and reporting of data regarding antibiotic drugs sold and distributed for use in food-producing animals.

Milestones

Within one year:

- FDA will publish enhanced annual summary reports on the sale and distribution of antibiotics approved for use in food-producing animals. An FDA summary report for 2009-2013 will provide baseline information regarding antibiotic sales for the period preceding the implementation of FDA Guidance for Industry #213.
- FDA will publish a proposed regulation that includes additional proposed reporting requirements for sponsors of antibiotics approved for use in food-producing animals.

Sub-Objective 2.4.3

Implement voluntary monitoring of antibiotic use and resistance in pre-harvest settings to provide nationally representative data while maintaining producer confidentiality.

Milestones

Within one year:

- USDA and FDA will seek public input on a plan for collecting drug use and resistance data on farms.

Within 3 years:

- CDC and FDA will work with EPA to evaluate the risk of environmental uses of antibiotics on human health.
- USDA and FDA will initiate collection of drug use and resistance data on farms. This information will be used to determine baselines and trends in drug use and resistance.

Sub-Objective 2.4.4

Collect quantitative data on antibiotic-resistance and management practices along various points at pre-harvest, harvest, and processing stages, in collaboration with producers and other stakeholders, and disseminate information as appropriate.

Milestones

Within one year:

- USDA will develop a plan for expanded monitoring of resistant bacteria throughout the food production continuum (e.g., pre-harvest, harvest, and processing of food products). On-farm sampling will be voluntary.

Within three years:

- USDA will implement collection of data on antibiotic-resistance and management practices during pre-harvest, harvest, and processing of food products. On-farm sampling will be voluntary. This information will be used to monitor trends in drug-resistant bacteria and identify potential mitigation strategies for further investigation.
- USDA will begin coordinated investigations of emerging zoonotic antibiotic resistant pathogens on the farm and at slaughter.

GOAL 3: ADVANCE DEVELOPMENT AND USE OF RAPID AND INNOVATIVE DIAGNOSTIC TESTS FOR IDENTIFICATION AND CHARACTERIZATION OF RESISTANT BACTERIA

Actions taken to achieve Goal 3 will fulfill:

Executive Order 13676, Section 8:
– *Promoting New and Next Generation Antibiotics and Diagnostics*

Provisions in **PCAST Recommendations #5 and #6** that concern:

– *International collaboration to promote diagnostic development*
– *Prizes for the development of breakthrough diagnostics*

Today's researchers are taking advantage of new technologies to develop rapid "point-of-need" diagnostic tests that can be used during a healthcare visit to distinguish between viral and bacterial infections and identify bacterial drug susceptibilities—an innovation that could significantly reduce unnecessary antibiotic use. The availability of new rapid diagnostic tests, combined with ongoing use of culture-based assays to identify new resistance mechanisms, will advance the detection and control of resistant bacteria, including the priority pathogens listed in Table 1.

By 2020, significant outcomes of Goal 3 will include:

- Development and dissemination of authorized point-of-need diagnostic tests that rapidly distinguish between bacterial and viral infections.
- Validation of diagnostic tests that rapidly determine the antibiotic-resistance profiles of bacteria of public health concern (Table 1).

To advance these outcomes, HHS agencies will award a prize for development of a rapid diagnostic test that can improve treatment of drug-resistant infections and facilitate antibiotic stewardship.

Objectives

3.1. Develop and Validate New Diagnostics—Including Tests That Rapidly Distinguish Between Viral and Bacterial Pathogens and Tests That Detect Antibiotic-Resistance—That Can Be Implemented in a Wide Range of Settings

Federal departments and agencies will work with domestic and international partners to develop rapid diagnostic tests that can identify clinical illnesses that may benefit from treatment with antibiotics, detect invasive bacterial pathogens in blood, cerebrospinal fluid, synovial fluid, and urine, and provide information to guide decisions on treatment and control of CRE, *Neisseria gonorrhoeae*, and other multidrug-resistant organisms.

Within three years:

- NIH will fund at least five new projects aimed at the development of rapid diagnostics, including:
  - Point-of-need diagnostic tests that rapidly distinguish between bacterial and viral infections.

  - Tests that can rapidly determine the antibiotic-resistance profiles of resistant bacterial threats of high importance to public health (Table 3), including CRE, MRSA, and ceftriaxone resistant *N. gonorrhoeae.*
- The Assistant Secretary for Preparedness and Response (ASPR)/Biomedical Advanced Research and Development Authority (BARDA) will fund at least three new diagnostic development projects that involve next-generation sequencing, multiplex molecular assays, or other new technologies that shorten the time needed for reliable and accurate detection of drug resistance.
- NIH and ASPR/BARDA will establish a prize for development of a rapid diagnostic test that can improve treatment of drug-resistant infections and facilitate antibiotic stewardship.
- DOD will fund projects to develop:
  - A functional (phenotypic) antibiotic susceptibility test that provides results more quickly than conventional susceptibility tests. This project will be conducted in collaboration with CDC.
  - A set of assays that can characterize the drug-resistance profile of any bacterial isolate.
  - An innovative method for antibiotic susceptibility testing (AST) aimed at eliminating the need to perform AST in centralized microbiology laboratories and enabling rapid AST in non-traditional healthcare settings.
- DOD will also fund at least one project involving next-generation sequencing technologies or bioinformatics platforms or tools that can be leveraged to improve diagnostics for drug-resistant or multidrug resistant pathogens.

Within five years:

- At least one new diagnostic product, the development of which was facilitated by NIH or ASPR/ BARDA, will be submitted for FDA approval or clearance.
- NIH and ASPR/BARDA will manage and administer a prize contest (see above) for development of a rapid diagnostic test that can improve treatment of drug-resistant infections and facilitate antibiotic stewardship.

3.2. Expand the Availability and Use of Diagnostics to Improve Treatment of Antibiotic-Resistant Bacteria, Enhance Infection Control, and Facilitate Outbreak Detection and Response in Healthcare and Community Settings

FDA and CMS are working with industry partners to streamline development and uptake of new diagnostic tests and facilitate their use to improve patient treatment and achieve public health goals. A major aim of these efforts is to develop well-defined reimbursement policies and incentives that encourage routine use of diagnostics in clinical settings to distinguish between bacterial and viral infections and identify the antibiotic susceptibilities of bacteria.

FDA and CMS signed a Memorandum of Understanding (MOU) on June 18, 2010 that facilitates interagency efforts to streamline regulatory processes in ways that reduce costs and timelines. New projects include the **FDA-CMS Parallel Review**, a pilot program that permits concurrent (rather than sequential) product reviews by FDA and CMS (i.e., while FDA reviews pre-market submissions for approval or clearance of diagnostic tests, CMS determines whether the tests will be covered by Medicare). Other projects designed to facilitate innovation include:

- **FDA Entrepreneur in Residence Program,** which provides technical support to small businesses who may lack the expertise to navigate the FDA approval or clearance process.
- **FDA Medical Device Innovation Consortium,** a partnership between a nonprofit organization and FDA to advance medical device regulatory science. Members include representatives of organizations involved in:
    - Medical and/or medical device research, development, treatment, or education
    - Promotion of public health
    - Regulatory science
- **FDA Medical Device Reimbursement Task Force**, which is pilot-testing a formal process that allows a device company to request a pre-submission meeting with FDA staff and one or more third-party payers to discuss reimbursement issues.

Milestones

Within one year:

- FDA and CMS will evaluate the potential impact of innovative regulatory pathways currently under development to foster the development of diagnostic tests by addressing issues related to Medicare reimbursement and coding.

Within three years:

- HHS will establish a process that allows product developers to provide data to CMS for use in developing Interpretive Guidelines that facilitate the use of tests for patient treatment, hospital infection control, and reporting of cases of disease during outbreaks.

Within five years:

- HHS will issue technical assistance and education modules and materials that assist healthcare providers and health systems in using diagnostic tests to improve patient management, enhance hospital infection control, and facilitate outbreak detection and response.

GOAL 4. ACCELERATE BASIC AND APPLIED RESEARCH AND DEVELOPMENT FOR NEW ANTIBIOTICS, OTHER THERAPEUTICS, AND VACCINES

Actions taken to achieve Goal 4 will fulfill

- Executive Order 13676, Section 8:
  - Promoting New and Next Generation Antibiotics and Diagnostics.
- Provisions in PCAST Recommendations #3, #4, and #5:
  - Fundamental Research
  - Clinical Trials with New Antibiotics
  - The Federal Government should Significantly Increase Economic Incentives for Developing Urgently Needed Antibiotics

Antibiotics that lose their effectiveness for treating human disease through antibiotic-resistance must be replaced with new drugs; alternatives to antibiotics are also needed in veterinary medicine. The advancement of drug development requires intensified efforts to boost basic scientific research, attract greater private investment, and facilitate clinical trials of new antibiotics. These activities are imperative to increase the number of antibiotic drug candidates in the drug-development pipeline. Goal 4 activities will also advance the discovery and development of other tools to combat resistance, including vaccines, alternatives to (or improved uses of) antibiotics in food animals, and non-traditional therapeutics to improve human health, including products that preserve or restore beneficial bacteria that live in human gastrointestinal tracts. By 2020, significant outcomes of Goal 4 will include:

- Characterization of the gut microbiome—the communities of microorganisms that live within the gastrointestinal tract—of at least one animal species raised for food. This outcome will help us understand how antibiotic treatments disrupt normal gut bacteria and how animal growth might be promoted—and bacterial diseases might be treated—without using antibiotics.
- Advancement of at least two new antibiotic drug candidates, non-traditional therapeutics, and/or vaccines from pre-clinical testing to clinical trials for treatment or prevention of human disease.
- Development of at least three new drug candidates or probiotic treatments as alternatives to antibiotics for promoting growth or preventing disease in animals.
- Creation of a biopharmaceutical incubator—a consortium of academic, biotechnology and pharmaceutical industry partners—to promote innovation and increase the number of antibiotics and antibodies in the drug-development pipeline.

OBJECTIVES

4.1. Conduct Research to Enhance Understanding of Environmental Factors That Facilitate the Development of Antibiotic-Resistance and the Spread of Resistance Genes That Are Common to Animals and Humans

Sub-Objective 4.1.1

Support basic research to exploit powerful new technologies, including systems biology, to advance the study of antibiotic-resistance and address the special problems posed by resistant Gram-negative pathogens such as CRE.

Milestones

Within one year:

- FDA, USDA, CDC, and NIH will host a roundtable of private and public sector experts to gather input on strategies to advance collaborative research to develop tools to combat antibiotic resistance using systems biology and other new technologies.

Within three years:

- A National Institute of Mathematical and Biological Synthesis (NIMBioS) working group will develop an analytic modeling framework for assessing the relationship between antibiotic use in livestock (measured at the population level) and the development of antibiotic resistance.

On an annual basis:

- HHS, NIH, FDA, USDA, CDC, DOD, and EPA will conduct a review to ensure that U.S. Government research resources are focused on high-priority antibiotic resistance issues (including basic research on the emergence and spread of resistance genes) and facilitate use of advanced technologies in research on antibiotic resistance (e.g., whole genome sequencing, proteomics, metagenomics, structural biology, bioinformatics).

Additional milestones related to basic research are provided under Objective 4.2.

Sub-Objective 4.1.2

Leverage existing partnerships, such as the NIH Antibacterial Resistance Leadership Group (ARLG), and international collaborations to reduce obstacles faced by pharmaceutical companies that are developing new antibiotics, other therapies, and vaccines. Partnerships will help identify human subjects qualified for enrollment in clinical trials of vaccines to prevent and antibiotics to treat resistant bacterial infections that occur sporadically, episodically, and/or in limited populations, generate and apply common clinical test protocols to multiple test groups of patients while sharing a common control group, and conduct other research-support activities as needed.

Milestones

Within one year:

- NIH will work with FDA and partners in industry and academia to:
    - Explore features necessary for developing a more robust clinical trials infrastructure for antibacterial product development.
    - Assess the feasibility of applying common clinical protocols for evaluation of multiple products while sharing a common control group. This approach may facilitate clinical testing of drugs to treat Gram-negative infections such as CRE that occur sporadically or episodically in limited populations (e.g., during hospital outbreaks).
- NIH will expand and strengthen the ARLG network, which facilitates clinical testing and validation of new antibacterial products and conducts studies to determine how existing products can be used in optimal ways to improve the treatment of resistant infections.
- FDA, USDA, CDC, and NIH will bring together experts in food production, agriculture, and public health to encourage collaborative research—from basic research to clinical testing—on antibiotic resistance.

Additional milestones related to fostering public/private partnerships and attracting greater private investment in antibiotics development are provided in Objective 4.6 and 4.7.

4.2. Increase Research Focused on Understanding the Nature of Microbial Communities, How Antibiotics Affect Them, and How They Can Be Harnessed to Prevent Disease

Milestones

Within three years:

- USDA, NIH, and CDC will support research on the spread of resistance genes between zoonotic pathogens and the commensal microbiota that live in the gastrointestinal tracts of animals and humans (i.e., in animal and human microbiomes).
- USDA, in consultation with NIH and CDC, will support research to map the gut microbiome of at least one food animal, using

metagenomic techniques and "big data" analysis tools. This research will advance understand antibiotic treatments disrupt the normal gut microbiome and how animal growth may be promoted without antibiotics. It may also suggest ways to treat bacterial animal diseases without using antibiotics.

4.3. Intensify Research and Development of New Therapeutics and New and Improved Vaccines, First-in-Class Drugs, and New Combination Therapies for Treatment of Bacterial Infections

Milestones

Within one year:

- The Chemical and Biological Defense Program/Defense Threat Reduction Agency (CBDP/DTRA) will:
  - Submit an Investigational New Drug (IND) application to FDA to initiate the clinical investigation of an antibiotic developed with DOD funding.
  - Award two new contracts to industry partners to accelerate advancement of novel small-molecule antibiotic therapies that circumvent known resistance mechanisms or potentiate the therapeutic efficacy of existing antibiotics (e.g., combination therapies). This activity will leverage ongoing efforts to develop treatments for infections caused by Select Agents (pathogens that might be used as biological weapons).

Within three years:

- NIH will arrange for clinical trials networks such as the Antibacterial Resistance Leadership Group (ARLG), (see Objective 4.1.2) to test a Gram-negative therapeutic agent with the goal of addressing use in a limited-population setting such as a hospital.
- NIH will launch a research program that uses systems biology to identify new drug targets that can be used to develop antibiotic drugs with new modes of action that make the development of resistance less likely.
- NIH will assist research partners who are developing novel classes of antibacterial drugs in submitting IND applications to FDA.

Within five years:

- NIH will support initial testing and validation of two new products (antibacterial drugs, novel therapeutics, or vaccines) to treat or prevent multidrug resistant Gram-negative pathogens. Once validated, these products will be transitioned to ASPR/BARDA or pharmaceutical companies for advanced development, including clinical efficacy trials (see also Objective 4.4).
- CBDP/DTRA will complete pre-clinical testing of an additional antibiotic drug and will support clinical trials of two new products to treat infections with Select Agents.

Additional milestones related to development of vaccines and combination therapies to address antibiotic resistance are provided under Objective 4.4.

4.4. Develop Non-Traditional Therapeutics, Vaccines, and Innovative Strategies to Minimize Outbreaks Caused by Resistant Bacteria in Human and Animal Populations

The development of non-traditional approaches that are less likely to drive resistance is an important step in breaking the cycle of drug development immediately followed by the development of resistance.

Examples of non-traditional therapeutic strategies include:

- Targeting bacterial virulence factors to prevent disease without killing bacteria.
- Using phage and phage-derived lysins to kill specific bacteria while preserving the microbiota.
- Creating vaccines that prevent infection with drug-resistant pathogens.
- Creating therapeutic products involving monoclonal or polyclonal antibodies.
- Developing products that restore or preserve beneficial bacteria in human and animal micro-biomes and prevent colonization with harmful bacteria (e.g., probiotics, prebiotics, or synthetic microbiota).
- Identifying natural compounds with antibiotic activity (e.g., phytochemicals, essential oils, organic acids, animal-derived lytic enzymes, and small interfering RNAs).

- Developing combination therapies and dosing strategies that slow the emergence of resistance.

Milestones: Therapeutics and Strategies for Use in Humans

Within one year:

- NIH will fund new projects to support the discovery and development of new types of antibacterial products (e.g., monoclonal antibodies, vaccines, or microbiota-based therapeutics), as well as adjunctive therapies to restore the activity of existing antibiotic drugs.
- DOD will implement laboratory use of new microfluidic technologies to detect antibodies that inhibit antibiotic-resistant bacteria.
- DOD will award:
    - Two new contracts focused on development of non-traditional therapeutics that are less likely to lead to the development of resistance (e.g., immunomodulators, therapeutic antibodies, or host-directed therapies).
    - Two new contracts focused on evaluating drug combinations that may decrease the emergence of drug resistance.
    - Two new contracts to explore revitalization and/or reformulation of antibacterial drug candidates that have failed to enter preclinical or clinical development due to undesirable characteristics related to solubility, pharmacokinetics, or toxicity.

Within three years:

- NIH, with guidance from FDA, will support development and evaluation of novel approaches for treatment of drug-resistant infections.
- DOD will investigate genes encoding antibodies that target drug-resistant bacteria and might be used in immunoprophylactic treatments.

Within five years:

- NIH will support the identification of alternative dosing strategies (e.g., combination therapies and shortened durations) that improve treatment for two bacterial pathogens of public health concern.
- NIH will launch clinical trials for two new products to treat or prevent high-priority bacterial pathogens and transition them to ASPR/BARDA or pharmaceutical companies for advanced development.
- Scientists at the Walter Reed Army Institute of Research will transition one antibiotic drug candidate to advanced development.

Milestones: Therapeutics and Strategies for Use in ANIMALS

Within one year:

- USDA, in collaboration with NIH, FDA, and the agriculture industry, will develop a research and development strategy to promote understanding of antibiotic-resistance and the creation of alternatives to (or improved uses of) antibiotics in food animals.
- USDA will solicit proposals that comprehensively develop research and outreach programs targeting development of novel alternatives to antibiotics for use in animals.

Within three years:

- USDA-funded research teams will develop three candidate alternatives to antibiotics used for promoting growth in animals (e.g., drugs or probiotic treatments) that do not disrupt the normal flora of the gut of food animals and enhance animal immune systems and resistance to disease.

Within five years:

- USDA-funded research teams will develop non-traditional alternatives to antibiotics that can be used (alone or in combination with existing antibiotics) to treat at least three priority bacterial pathogens of livestock and poultry.
- USDA-supported researchers will study genes that confer resistance to high-priority agricultural animal diseases (e.g., Bovine Respiratory Disease Complex) to facilitate genetic selection for animals with less susceptibility to infections whose treatments typically require significant use of antibiotics.

4.5. Expand Ongoing Efforts to Provide Key Data and Materials to Support the Development of Promising Antibacterial Drug Candidates and Promising Vaccines That Can Reduce the Need to Treat Bacterial Infections

CARB Economic Incentives Working Group

Economic incentives for product development are critical to ensuring diverse and robust pipeline of antibiotics. The PCAST report provides several key recommendations on economic incentives.

In response to these recommendations, the Office of Science and Technology Policy (OSTP) and National Security Council (NSC) staff of the

Executive Office of the President convened a working group to conduct an analysis of these potential economic incentives. Efforts to attract more private investment will reflect the recommendations of the CARB Economic Incentives Working Group.

Milestones

Within one year:

- NIH and ASPR/BARDA will implement a strategy for assisting research partners who are developing novel classes of antibacterial drugs in fulfilling the requirements of FDA IND applications.
- NIH and ASPR/BARDA will meet on a semi-annual basis with investigators who participate in the Antibiotic Resistance Biopharmaceutical Incubator (see Objective 4.7) to evaluate progress in providing technical resources for *in vitro* and *in vivo* screening of resistant pathogens of public health concern.
- Agencies with existing capabilities will ensure that genomic sequence data, proteomic data, and other related AR data sets generated with U.S. Government funding will be made publically available in a manner consistent with protecting personally identifiable information.
- DOD will develop three specimen panels as a critical resource for evaluating the efficacy of novel antibiotic therapies against multidrug-resistant Select Agents. The panels will include: (1) resistant bacterial isolates suitable for work in lower-level (BSL-2) biocontainment laboratories, (2) multidrug resistant strains of Select Agents, and (3) attenuated strains of multidrug resistant Select Agents. The panels will be maintained within DOD and will be available through the Select Agent Core Antibiotic Screening Program.

Within three years:

- NIH and ASPR/BARDA will identify at least twelve candidate products for preclinical development support and support three candidate products from preclinical development through IND submission (see also Objective 4.4).

Within five years:

- All agencies will ensure that genomic sequence data, proteomic data, and other related AR data sets generated with U.S. Government funding will be made publicly available in a manner consistent with protecting personally identifiable information.

4.6. Enhance Opportunities for Public-Private Partnerships to Accelerate Research on New Antibiotics and Other Tools to Combat Resistant Bacteria

HHS is partnering with pharmaceutical and biotechnology companies to advance the development of antibiotics through a "portfolio approach" in which companies investigate multiple drug candidates at the same time. This approach balances risk (for the companies and the government) by increasing the likelihood that one or more drug candidates will advance from preclinical testing to commercial use.

Milestones

Within one year:

- The HHS Public Health Emergency Medical Countermeasures Enterprise (PHEMCE) will ensure coordination with the U.S. Task Force for Combating Antibiotic-Resistant in promoting public-private partnerships to develop new and next-generation countermeasures to target antibiotic-resistant bacteria that present a serious or urgent threat to public health.
- ASPR/BARDA will create at least one additional portfolio partnership with a pharmaceutical or biotechnology company to accelerate development of antibacterial drugs.

Within three years:

- At least two antibiotic drugs developed by portfolio partners for treatment of an urgent or serious pathogen (Table 1) will enter Phase III clinical investigation.

Within five years:

- IND applications for at least two additional antibiotic drugs developed by portfolio partners will be submitted for FDA approval.

4.7. Create a Biopharmaceutical Incubator—A Consortium of Academic, Biotechnology and Pharmaceutical Industry Partners—To Promote Innovation and Increase the Number of Antibiotics in the Drug-Development Pipeline

ASPR/BARDA, in collaboration with NIH, will establish a pharmaceutical incubator that brings inventors and researchers together with start-up companies to explore creative ideas that could lead to the development of new antibiotics or non-traditional therapies. Like the ARLG network described in Objective 4.1.2 and the "portfolio partnerships" described in Objective 4.6, the biopharmaceutical incubator will help attract greater private investment by reducing the risks and obstacles faced by drug companies who are developing new antibiotics.

Milestones

Within one year:

- ASPR/BARDA and NIH will work with a consortium of industry partners to develop a strategy for establishing the Antibiotic Resistance Biopharmaceutical Incubator (ARBI).

Within three years:

- The ARBI will be operational, with technical services in place to facilitate toxicology studies, animal challenge studies, and other activities needed to accelerate drug development.

On an annual basis:

- ASPR/BARDA and NIH will assess progress in meeting ARBI's five-year goals: identifying at least five targets for novel therapeutics, generating *in vivo* data to validate at least three of these targets, generating at least three antibacterial drug candidates, and transitioning at least two of these candidates from preclinical testing to submission of an FDA IND application to begin clinical trials.

GOAL 5. IMPROVE INTERNATIONAL COLLABORATION AND CAPACITIES FOR ANTIBIOTIC - RESISTANCE PREVENTION, SURVEILLANCE, CONTROL, AND ANTIBIOTIC RESEARCH AND DEVELOPMENT

Actions taken to achieve Goal 5 will fulfill

- Executive Order 13676, Section 9:
  - *International Cooperation*
- Provisions in PCAST Recommendation #8:
  - *Ensure Effective International Coordination*

Antibiotic resistance is a global problem that requires global solutions. The United States, led by the Secretaries of State, USDA, and HHS and the Administrator of USAID, will engage in international action with foreign ministries of health and agriculture, the World Health Organization (WHO), the Food and Agriculture Organization of the United Nations (FAO), the World Organization for Animal Health (OIE), and other domestic and international stakeholders to strengthen national and international capacities to detect, monitor, analyze, and report antibiotic resistance, provide resources and incentives to spur the development of therapeutics and diagnostics for use in humans and animals, and strengthen regional networks and global partnerships that help prevent and control the emergence and spread of resistance. The United States will support the development of the *WHO Global Action Plan on Antimicrobial Resistance,* strengthen cooperation under the European Union-United States Trans-Atlantic Task Force on Antimicrobial Resistance (TATFAR), promote antibiotic resistance as an international health priority, and mobilize resources for global activities through bilateral, regional, and multilateral venues such as the Global Health Security Agenda.

By 2020, significant outcomes of Goal 5 will include:

- Elevation of antibiotic resistance as an international priority for global health and security.
- Enhanced capacity to identify antimicrobial-resistant pathogens in more than fifteen partner countries.
- Establishment of a common U.S.- European Union (EU) system for sharing and analyzing bacterial resistance patterns for priority pathogens.

- Development of a global database to collect harmonized quantitative data on the use of antibacterial agents in animals.
- Development of national plans to combat antibiotic resistance and improve antibiotic stewardship in low- and middle-income countries.
- Strengthened regulatory and supply chain systems that assure the quality, safety, and efficacy of antibiotics used in low- and middle-income countries.

OBJECTIVES

Surveillance: Establish capacity to detect, analyze, and report antibiotic resistance, in order to make available information needed for evidence-based decision making in individual countries and globally.

5.1. Promote Laboratory Capability to Identify at Least Three of the Seven WHO Priority Antimicrobial Resistant (AMR) Pathogens[5] Using Standardized, Reliable Detection Assays

The WHO AMR Pathogens and types of resistance of concern include:

- *Escherichia coli:* resistance to 3rd generation cephalosporins and to fluoroquinolones
- *Klebsiella pneumoniae:* resistance to 3rd generation cephalosporins and to carbapenems
- *Staphylococcus aureus:* methicillin resistance, or MRSA
- *Streptococcus pneumoniae:* resistance (non-susceptibility) to penicillin
- *Non-typhoidal Salmonella (NTS):* resistance to fluoroquinolones
- *Shigella species:* resistance to fluoroquinolones
- *Neisseria gonorrhoeae:* reduced susceptibility to 3rd generation cephalosporins

Milestones

Within one year:

- CDC and USAID will work with ministries of health in at least twelve to fifteen countries to complete laboratory proficiency assessments, and will assess expansion of bilateral relationships to additional countries.
- DOD will work with international partner laboratories to identify and enhance local proficiency and capabilities and will conduct assessments on an annual basis.

Within three years:

- CDC and USAID will provide technical assistance to foreign ministries of health on developing national plans for strengthening laboratory-based surveillance for antimicrobial resistance, and will complete assessments of laboratory capacity in additional counties.

Within five years:

- Public health laboratories in at least fifteen partner countries will be able to identify at least three of the seven WHO priority AMR pathogens and will report their results to WHO, to international surveillance networks, and—in the case of a public health emergency of international concern—to International Health Regulations (IHR) focal points.

5.2. Collaborate with WHO, OIE, and Other International Efforts Focused on the Development of Integrated, Laboratory-Based Surveillance to Detect and Monitor Antibiotic Resistance in Relevant Animal and Human Foodborne Pathogens

Milestones

Within one year:

- USDA, FDA, and CDC will develop a plan, in partnership with WHO, the Pan American Health Organization, and other international organizations to identify key partner laboratories that conduct AMR testing of animal foodborne pathogens.

Within three years:

- USDA and FDA, in conjunction with CDC and international partners, will:
  - Develop a process for assessing national and regional capabilities for surveillance of antibiotic resistance in animal and human foodborne pathogens.
  - Identify challenges to harmonizing AMR data requirements and collection methods on an international scale.
  - Assess the current status of national capabilities for molecular diagnostics and epidemiology and address the need for access to these capacities.
  - Identify additional partners who can assess laboratory testing proficiencies and provide training for technology transfer.
  - Work with regional partners to monitor the emergence and spread of resistance genes in animal and foodborne pathogens on an ongoing basis, using molecular techniques.
  - Expand activities conducted through other USG-funded activities (e.g., the Asia-Pacific Economic Cooperation) to inventory existing worldwide laboratory resources and assess the need for national and regional improvements to support surveillance for drug-resistant animal and human foodborne pathogens. These efforts will include expansion of training opportunities in pathogen characterization and diagnostics.
- DOD will develop a scalable, evidence-based database of global information on antimicrobial resistance and issue annual reports of findings.

Within five years:

- USDA, FDA, and CDC will initiate regional collaborations to monitor the emergence and spread of resistance genes in food, animal, and human foodborne pathogens, using genome sequencing techniques.
- USDA and FDA will work with CDC and international partners to provide training in laboratory methodologies (in-country or within the U.S.) and initiate collaborations to promote training as opportunities arise.
- USDA, FDA, and CDC will work through existing laboratory and public health networks—such as PulseNet International and the Red Interamericana de Laboratorios de Análisis de Alimentos (RILAA)—to transfer technology and train local partners.

5.3. Develop a Mechanism for International Communication of Critical Events That May Signify New Resistance Trends with Global Public and Animal Health Implications

Milestones:

Within one year:

- CDC will work with TATFAR partners to develop a common U.S.-E.U. system for sharing and analyzing bacterial resistance patterns for pathogens identified as urgent and serious threats in Table 1.
- HHS/OGA, USDA, FDA and CDC will work with TATFAR partners to address TATFAR Recommendation #18, which calls for the formation of an international working group to identify key knowledge gaps about transmission of drug-resistant bacteria in animals and the use of antibiotics in animal agriculture.

Within three years:

- CDC will work with WHO and other partners to develop a secure website for real-time sharing of international surveillance data on antimicrobial resistance in order to facilitate early warning and notification of significant events to WHO, regional and international disease surveillance networks (e.g., European Centre for Disease Prevention and Control), and IHR. These efforts will make use of data-sharing practices developed by the U.S. and TATFAR (see above). Steps include developing terms of reference, assessing IT requirements, and identifying mechanisms for validating and sharing information.
- CDC will deploy the website in partnership with the international community and will help test, monitor, evaluate, and improve its utility.
- USDA will identify next steps in addressing knowledge gaps about development and spread of antibiotic resistance in animals, based on the conclusions of the work group formed in fulfillment of TATFAR Recommendation #18 (see above).

Within five years:

- CDC and other U.S. agencies will help ensure access to—and full participation by—public health authorities in all WHO member countries.

- USDA will engage TATFAR and other regional partners in sharing information about drug-resistance trends with implications for animal health.

5.4. Promote the Generation and Dissemination of Information Needed to Effectively Address Antibiotic-Resistance

Sub-Objective 5.4.1

Support consistent international standards for determining whether bacteria are resistant to antibiotics.

Milestones

Within one year:

- U.S. agencies, led by CDC and USAID, will engage stakeholders in establishing harmonized definitions of drug resistance for surveillance purposes (e.g., by standardizing interpretive criteria for analyzing the results of antibiotic susceptibility tests).
- As part of these efforts, DOD will continue to engage and support existing and newly-identified international partners through sharing of technological packages for surveillance and reporting purposes.

Within three years:

- U.S. agencies, led by CDC, will work with the six WHO regional surveillance networks to implement harmonized definitions of resistance for surveillance programs integrating data on WHO and CDC priority pathogens.

Sub-Objective 5.4.2

Develop international collaborations to gather country-specific and regional information on drivers of antibiotic resistance, identify evidence-based interventions, adapt these strategies to new settings, and evaluate their effectiveness.

Within one year:

- U.S. agencies, led by the Department of State and HHS, will develop a strategy for working with partner countries to elevate the issue of antibiotic resistance as an international priority for global health security.

- U.S. agencies, led by HHS/OGA, will support development of the *WHO Global Action Plan on Antimicrobial Resistance.* As part of this effort, U.S. agencies will support the inclusion of provisions that require open access to research data on factors that drive the emergence of resistance and strategies to prevent its spread.

Within three years:

- The Department of State, HHS, and other agency partners will convene a group of international stakeholders to discuss best practices for research collaborations on antimicrobial resistance, including methodologies, data-sharing policies, management plans and interoperability.
- U.S. agencies will work with WHO, FAO, and OIE to support implementation of the *WHO Global Action Plan on Antimicrobial Resistance* by:
    - Assessing country-specific and regional factors that drive the development of antimicrobial resistance, building on existing risk management frameworks such as the Codex Alimentarius.
    - Establishing a global database to collect harmonized quantitative data on the use of antibacterial agents in animals.
    - Forging partnerships aimed at reducing the use of medically-important antibiotics for growth promotion in food animals.

Over five years:

- The Department of State, HHS, and other agency partners will continue to promote antibiotic resistance as an international health priority by raising the issue of antibiotic resistance during bilateral consultations and multilateral forums and by advancing implementation of the Global Health Security Agenda (GHSA) Antimicrobial Resistance Action Package.

Sub-Objective 5.4.3

Provide technical assistance as needed to underdeveloped and developing nations to improve their capacity to detect and respond effectively to antibiotic resistance.

Milestones

Within three years:

- CDC will develop bilateral agreements with twelve to fifteen countries to develop country-specific surveillance strategies, and will assess expansion of these activities to additional countries (see also Objective 5.1).
- CDC and other U.S. agencies will assist partner countries with development and implementation of national strategies for infection prevention and control in healthcare facilities.

Within five years:

CDC and other U.S. agencies will assist at least fifteen countries with collection of resistance surveillance data and data-sharing with stakeholders.

Research and Development: Incentivize development of therapeutics and diagnostics for humans and animals.

5.5. Establish and Promote International Collaboration and Public-Private Partnerships to Incentivize Development of New Therapeutics to Counter Antibiotic Resistance, Including New, Next-Generation, and Other Alternatives to Antibiotics, Vaccines, and Affordable, Rapidly Deployable, Point-of-Need Diagnostics

Milestones

Within one year:

- U.S. agencies, led by HHS, will work with WHO, FAO, OIE, and other international partners to accelerate investment in research to develop point-of-care diagnostics, vaccines, and drugs to combat resistant bacteria, as well as to investigate the microbiomes of food animals. For example, U.S. agencies and partners in industry and academia will work with TATFAR partners to advance collaborations with EU nations to facilitate translational and clinical research on tools to slow the emergence and spread of antimicrobial resistance. U.S. agencies will also explore collaborations with the New Drugs 4 Bad Bugs (ND4BB) programs of the Innovative Medicines Initiative.

Within three years:

- U.S. agencies and partners in industry and academia will establish or expand additional international partnerships to advance research to reduce antibacterial resistance through the development of point-of-care diagnostics, vaccines, and drugs.
- USDA will establish or expand five collaborative international partnerships to facilitate research regarding development of alternatives to antibiotics, as well as vaccines and new antimicrobial drugs that are less likely to develop resistance.

Prevention and Control: Strengthen systems in countries, regional networks, and global partnerships to prevent and control the emergence and spread of antibiotic resistance through evidence-based interventions, and monitor and evaluate the effectiveness of interventions.

5.6. Support Countries to Develop and Implement National Plans to Combat Antibiotic Resistance and Strategies to Enhance Antimicrobial Stewardship

Milestones

Within one year:

- U.S. agencies, led by HHS/OGA, will collaborate with the global community to ensure that the *WHO Global Action Plan on Antimicrobial Resistance* incorporates approaches and interventions that benefit all healthcare programs and calls for the development of national plans to combat antibiotic resistance (see also Sub-Objective 5.4.2).

Within three years:

- CDC and USAID will provide technical assistance to foreign ministries of health and agriculture to advance the use of tools and interventions that have proven successful at slowing the spread of resistance in healthcare and agricultural settings (e.g., infection prevention and control and antibiotic stewardship programs in hospitals).
- U.S. agencies, led by USAID and CDC, will support at least four Low and Middle Income Countries (LMICs) in developing and/or operationalizing national antimicrobial resistance containment plans,

national healthcare-facility infection prevention and control plans, antimicrobial stewardship strategies, or comparable packages of interventions.

Within five years:

- U.S. agencies, led by USAID and CDC, will:
  - Support at least three additional LMICs in developing and/or operationalizing national antimicrobial resistance containment plans, national healthcare facility infection prevention and control plans, antimicrobial stewardship strategies, or comparable packages of interventions.
  - Support the implementation of national infection prevention and control programs in at least twenty priority healthcare facilities in eight LMICs.
  - Support operational research that leads to remedial actions and improved antibiotic use in at least eight healthcare facilities in 4 LMICs.
  - Develop and disseminate at least four global technical leadership documents/reports for use by LMICs and the global community, that review approaches, results, lessons learned, and recommendations related to key antibiotic containment strategies.
- U.S. agencies, led by HHS/OGA, the Department of State and USAID, will support international advocacy and coordination to contain the common threat of antimicrobial resistance, through collaboration with WHO and other partners and participation in multilateral forums, such as the 4th Conference on Improving Use of Medicines (ICIUM).
- USDA will use Veterinary Accreditation training modules—including the Judicious Use Module —to assist countries in at least three WHO regions in developing sustainable veterinary service capacity to monitor and slow antibiotic resistance and to report outbreaks of drug resistant disease to WHO, international surveillance networks, collaborative reporting structures, or (when appropriate) to International Health Regulations (IHR) focal points.
- USDA will translate the Judicious Use Module into three other languages.

A milestone on development of national plans for strengthening laboratory-based surveillance for antibiotic resistance is provided under Objective 5.1.

5.7. Partner with Other Nations to Promote Quality, Safety, and Efficacy of Antibiotics and Strengthen Their Pharmaceutical Supply Chains

Milestones

Within three years:

- U.S. agencies, led by USAID, will support country systems to enhance access to and appropriate use of quality-assured, safe, effective essential antibiotics through improved medicines, regulatory capacity and quality assurance systems, modern procurement practices, reliable and secure supply chains, and equitable pharmaceutical services in at least four LMICs.

Within five years:

- U.S. agencies, led by USAID, will:
  - Support country systems that enhance access to quality-assured, safe, effective essential antibiotics in at least eight LMICs.
  - Develop and disseminate at least four global technical leadership documents/reports, for use by LMICs and the global community, that review approaches, results, lessons learned, and recommendations on access to quality-assured, safe, effective antibiotics and issues related to regulation, quality assurance, and patient safety in the use of antibiotics.

5.8. Coordinate Regulatory Approaches by Collaborating with International Organizations Such As FAO and OIE to Harmonize International Data Submission Requirements and Risk Assessment Guidelines Related to the Licensure and/or Approval of Veterinary Medicinal Products, Including Antibacterial Agents, Vaccines, and Diagnostics, to the Extent Possible

U.S. agencies are working in partnership with TATFAR, the WHO Advisory Group on Integrated Surveillance of Antimicrobial Resistance (AGISAR), the International Conference on Harmonization of Technical Requirements for Registration of Pharmaceuticals for Human Use (ICH), the International Cooperation on Harmonization of Technical Requirements for

Veterinary Medicinal Products (VICH), the Institute for International Cooperation in Animal Biologics (IICAB), and the International Medical Device Regulators Forum (IMDRF) to facilitate the development of antibacterial drugs for human and agricultural use, diagnostic tests for human and animal bacterial diseases, vaccines for human and animal bacterial diseases, and risk assessments on the use of medically-important antibacterial drugs in agriculture.

Milestones

Within one year:

- FDA and USDA will contribute to and participate in global or regional cooperation with international organizations, including AGISAR, VICH, IICAB, and IMDRF, regarding development of vaccines, antibacterial drugs, and diagnostic tests for use in agriculture, and regarding risk assessments of the use of medically-important antibiotics in agriculture.
- USDA will maintain the U.S. commitment to VICH and IICAB, expanding the Global Outreach Forum to:
    - Promote the use of VICH guidance for safety, quality, potency and effective use of vaccines outside of the three cooperating major regions (the U.S., Japan, and the European Union).
    - Facilitate input from a broadened base of participating countries and economies.
- USDA will plan and participate in at least three VICH Global Outreach Forums over the first two years.
- USDA will hold at least one international meeting in collaboration with IICAB to discuss U.S. regulatory policy in a workshop setting.

Within three years:

- FDA and USDA will consult with regional health authorities about their processes for achieving regulatory approval of new antibacterial drugs, diagnostics, and vaccines for use in medicine and agriculture and for conducting risk assessments on the use of medically-important antibiotics in agriculture.

Within five years:

- FDA and USDA will engage China and additional interested partner countries to exchange technical information and harmonize approaches for risk assessment and regulation of veterinary medicinal products.

- FDA and USDA will work with OIE and other international partners on development of standardized methods of reporting antimicrobial drug use in animals.

APPENDIX

Table 3. CDC's Antibiotic-Resistant Threats in the United States, 2013

URGENT Threat Level Pathogens (3)
Clostridium difficile
250,000 infections per year requiring hospitalization or affecting hospitalized patients
14,000 deaths per year
At least $1 Billion in excess medical costs per year
C. difficile deaths increased 400% between 2000-2007 because of the emergence of a strain resistant to a common antibiotic class (fluoroquinolones)
Almost half of infections occur in people younger than 65, but more than 90% of deaths occur in people 65 and older
Half of C. difficile infections first show symptoms in hospitalized or recently hospitalized patients, and half show symptoms in nursing home patients or in people recently cared for in doctors' offices and clinics who received antibiotics
The majority (71%) of pediatric Clostridium difficile infections, which are bacterial infections that cause severe diarrhea and are potentially life-threatening, occur among children in the general community, 73% were found to have recently taken antibiotics prescribed in doctor's offices for other outpatient settings[6]
Carbapenem-Resistant Enterobacteriaceae*
Out of ~140,000 healthcare-associated Enterobacteriaceae infections per year, more than 9,000 are caused by CRE (7,900
CR-Klebsiella spp; 1,400 CR-E coli)
Out of ~140,000 healthcare-associated Enterobacteriaceae infections per year, more than 9,000 are caused by CRE (7,900
CR-Klebsiella spp; 1,400 CR-E coli)
44 States have had at least one type of CRE confirmed by CDC testing
CRE are resistant to nearly all antibiotics including carbapenems—the antibiotic of last resort
Neisseria gonorrhoeae **(Notifiable to CDC)**
Neisseria gonorrhoeae causes gonorrhea, is the second most common reportable infection in the United States, and is developing resistance to the cephalosporin antibiotics, the last line treatment option for this infection

Table 3. (Continued)

Of the 820,000 cases per year, 30% (246,000) now demonstrate resistance to at least one antibiotic
If cephalosporin-resistant N. gonorrhoeae becomes widespread, the public health impact during a 10-year period is estimated to be 75,000 additional cases of pelvic inflammatory disease, 15,000 cases of epididymitis, and 222 additional HIV infections, with an estimated direct medical cost of at least $235 million
SERIOUS Threat Level Pathogens (12)
Multidrug-Resistant Acinetobacter
12,000 healthcare-associated Acinetobacter infections occur in the U S of which 7,000 are multidrug-resistant ~ 500 deaths per year
At least three different classes of antibiotics no longer cure resistant Acinetobacter infections
Drug-Resistant Campylobacter
Campylobacter causes ~1 3 Million infections, 13, 000 hospitalizations and 120 deaths each year; 310,000 (25%) drug-resistant Campylobacter infections are found each year
Campylobacter drug resistance increased from 13% in 1997 to 25% in 2011
Campylobacter spreads from animals to people through contaminated food, particularly raw or undercooked chicken and unpasteurized milk
Antibiotic use in food animals can results in resistant Campylobacter than can spread to humans
Fluconazole-Resistant Candida
Out of 46,000 Candida yeast infections per year, 3,400 (30%) of patients with bloodstream infections with drug-resistant (DR)-Candida die during their hospitalization
CDC estimates that each case of Candida infection results in 3-13 days of additional hospitalization and a total of $6,000-$29,000 in direct healthcare costs per patient

SERIOUS Threat Level Pathogens (12
Extended Spectrum β-Lactamase (ESBL) Producing Enterobacteriaceae*
Extended Spectrum β-Lactamase (ESBL) is an enzyme that allows bacteria to become resistant to a wide spectrum of penicillins and cephalosporins
Of 140,000 Enterobacteriaceae infections per year, 26,000 are drug resistant causing 1,700 deaths
26,000 healthcare-associated Enterobacteriaceae infections are caused by ESBL-Enteorbacteriaceae
26,000 healthcare-associated Enterobacteriaceae infections are caused by ESBL-Enteorbacteriaceae
Vancomycin-Resistant Enterococcus
Of 66,000 Enterococcus infections per year, 20,000 are drug resistant causing 1,300 deaths
Enterococcus strains resistant to vancomycin leave few or no treatment options
Multidrug-Resistant Pseudomonas aeruginosa

Of 51,000 Pseudomonas infections per year, 6,700 are multidrug resistant causing 440 deaths
13% of severe healthcare-associated infections caused by Pseudomonas are multidrug resistant, meaning nearly all or all antibiotics no longer cure these infections
Drug-Resistant Non-Typhoidal Salmonella* (Notifiable to CDC)
Non-typhoidal Salmonella causes 1 2 million infections per year, of which 100,000 are drug-resistant resulting in 23,000 hospitalizations and 450 deaths each year
Non-typhoidal Salmonella results in higher number of hospital stays, length of stay, and treatment costs
Drug-Resistant Salmonella typhi (Notifiable to CDC)
Of 21 7 M Salmonella typhi infections worldwide, 5,700 illnesses in the U S with 3,800 (67%) of infections are drug-resistant resulting in 620 hospitalizations each year
Before the antibiotic era or in areas where antibiotics are unavailable, Salmonella typhi results in up to 20% deaths
Drug-Resistant Shigella* (Notifiable to CDC)
Shigella causes ~ 500,000 illnesses, 5,500 hospitalizations, and 40 deaths each year in the U S
Since 2006, Shigella resistance to traditional first-line antibiotics has become so high that physicians must now rely on alternative drugs (ciprofloxacin and azithromycin) to treat infections
Methicillin-Resistant Staphylococcus aureus (MRSA)*
Over 80,000 invasive MRSA infections and 11,285 related deaths per year (in 2011)
Severe MRSA infections most commonly occur during or soon after inpatient medical care
Between 2005 and 2001, overall rates of invasive MRSA dropped 31% predominantly due to appropriate medical procedures implemented in central-line maintenance
Drug-Resistant Streptococcus pneumoniae* (Notifiable to CDC)
Of 4 million disease incidents and 22,000 deaths; 1 2 M are drug resistant (to amoxicillin and azithromycin (Z-Pak) resulting in 19,000 excess hospitalizations and 7,900 deaths
In 30% of S. pneumoniae cases, the bacteria are fully resistant to one or more antibiotics causing complications in treatment and death
Pneumococcal pneumonia accounts for 72% of all direct medical costs for treatment of pneumococcal disease and in excess of $96 million in medical costs per year
Pneumococcal conjugate vaccine (PCV) prevents disease, reduces antibiotic-resistance by blocking the transmission of resistant S. pneumoniae strains, and protects against 13 strains of Streptococcus

SERIOUS Threat Level Pathogens (12)
Drug-Resistant Tuberculosis* (Notifiable to CDC)
Tuberculosis is among the most common infectious diseases and cause of death worldwide
Of 10,528 Tb cases in the U S in 2011, 1,042 (9 9%) were resistant to antibiotics resulting in 50 deaths
CDC manages 5 Tb Regional Training and Medical Consultation Centers (RTMCCs) and ongoing surveillance for drug-resistant Tb in all 50 states and DC using the National Tuberculosis Surveillance System (NTSS)
OF CONCERN Threat Level Pathogens (3)
Vancomycin-Resistant Staphylococcus aureas (Notifiable to CDC)
Few cases thus far (13 cases in 4 States since 2002)
Staph a strains resistant to vancomycin leave very few or no treatment options
Erythromycin-Resistant Group A Streptococcus
Group A Strep (GAS) causes many illnesses including strep throat (up to 2 6 M cases per year), toxic shock syndrome, and "flesh-eating" disease (necrotizing fasciitis, 25-35% fatal)
Erythromycin-resistant GAS causes 1,300 illnesses and 160 deaths
Current concern is the increase in bacteria that show resistance to clindamycin—which has a unique role in treatment of GAS infections
Clindamycin-Resistant Group B Streptococcus
Of 27,000 Group B Strep (GBS) cases, 7,600 illnesses are drug-resistant resulting in 440 deaths in the U S each year

End Notes

1. The TB activities identified in the NAP are included as they represent critical near-term public health activities that will support progress to reduce the burden of drug-resistant TB in the U.S. Additional domestic and global activities to address drug-resistant TB will be provided in a companion action plan specific to TB and will be submitted to the President no later than September, 2015. The companion action plan will build on recommendations of the Federal TB Task Force (http://www.cdc.gov/mmwr/pdf/rr/rr5803.pdf) as well the work of the interagency USG TB working group.
2. The WHO priority AMR pathogens are a subset of the pathogens identified as urgent and serious threats in Table 3.
3. The ten EIP sites are: California, Colorado, Connecticut, Georgia, Maryland, Minnesota, New Mexico, New York, Oregon and Tennessee.
4. Cecal samples are taken from the large intestines of swine, cattle, and poultry. The cecum is a pouch at the beginning of the large intestine.
5. The WHO priority AMR pathogens are a subset of the pathogens identified as urgent and serious threats in Table 3.
6. Wendt, J.M. et al. *Clostridium difficile* Infection Among Children Across Diverse US Geographic Locations. *Pediatrics.* January 3, 2014.

In: National Strategy
Editor: Anthony Phillips
ISBN: 978-1-63483-072-0

Chapter 3

EXECUTIVE ORDER 13676: COMBATING ANTIBIOTIC-RESISTANT BACTERIA*

Barack Obama

By the authority vested in me as President by the Constitution and the laws of the United States of America, I hereby order as follows:

Section 1. Policy. The discovery of antibiotics in the early 20th century fundamentally transformed human and veterinary medicine. Antibiotics save millions of lives each year in the United States and around the world. The rise of antibiotic-resistant bacteria, however, represents a serious threat to public health and the economy. The Centers for Disease Control and Prevention (CDC) in the Department of Health and Human Services (HHS) estimates that annually at least two million illnesses and 23,000 deaths are caused by antibiotic-resistant bacteria in the United States alone.

Detecting, preventing, and controlling antibiotic resistance requires a strategic, coordinated, and sustained effort. It also depends on the engagement of governments, academia, industry, healthcare providers, the general public, and the agricultural community, as well as international partners. Success in this effort will require significant efforts to: minimize the emergence of antibiotic-resistant bacteria; preserve the efficacy of new and existing

* This is an edited, reformatted and augmented version of an Executive Order, issued by the White House Office of the Press Secretary, September 18, 2014.

antibacterial drugs; advance research to develop improved methods for combating antibiotic resistance and conducting antibiotic stewardship; strengthen surveillance efforts in public health and agriculture; develop and promote the use of new, rapid diagnostic technologies; accelerate scientific research and facilitate the development of new antibacterial drugs, vaccines, diagnostics, and other novel therapeutics; maximize the dissemination of the most up-to-date information on the appropriate and proper use of antibiotics to the general public and healthcare providers; work with the pharmaceutical industry to include information on the proper use of over-the-counter and prescription antibiotic medications for humans and animals; and improve international collaboration and capabilities for prevention, surveillance, stewardship, basic research, and drug and diagnostics development.

The Federal Government will work domestically and internationally to detect, prevent, and control illness and death related to antibiotic-resistant infections by implementing measures that reduce the emergence and spread of antibiotic-resistant bacteria and help ensure the continued availability of effective therapeutics for the treatment of bacterial infections.

Sec. 2. Oversight and Coordination. Combating antibiotic-resistant bacteria is a national security priority. The National Security Council staff, in collaboration with the Office of Science and Technology Policy, the Domestic Policy Council, and the Office of Management and Budget, shall coordinate the development and implementation of Federal Government policies to combat antibiotic-resistant bacteria, including the activities, reports, and recommendations of the Task Force for Combating Antibiotic-Resistant Bacteria established in section 3 of this order.

Sec. 3. Task Force for Combating Antibiotic-Resistant Bacteria. There is hereby established the Task Force for Combating Antibiotic-Resistant Bacteria (Task Force), to be co-chaired by the Secretaries of Defense, Agriculture, and HHS.

(a) Membership. In addition to the Co-Chairs, the Task Force shall consist of representatives from:

i. the Department of State;
ii. the Department of Justice;
iii. the Department of Veterans Affairs;
iv. the Department of Homeland Security;
v. the Environmental Protection Agency;
vi. the United States Agency for International Development;

vii. the Office of Management and Budget;
viii. the Domestic Policy Council;
ix. the National Security Council staff;
x. the Office of Science and Technology Policy;
xi. the National Science Foundation; and
xii. such executive departments, agencies, or offices as the Co-Chairs may designate.

Each executive department, agency, or office represented on the Task Force (Task Force agency) shall designate an employee of the Federal Government to perform the functions of the Task Force. In performing its functions, the Task Force may make use of existing interagency task forces on antibiotic resistance.

(b)Mission. The Task Force shall identify actions that will provide for the facilitation and monitoring of implementation of this order and the National Strategy for Combating Antibiotic-Resistant Bacteria (Strategy).

(c)Functions.

(i) By February 15, 2015, the Task Force shall submit a 5-year National Action Plan (Action Plan) to the President that outlines specific actions to be taken to implement the Strategy. The Action Plan shall include goals, milestones, and metrics for measuring progress, as well as associated timelines for implementation. The Action Plan shall address recommendations made by the President's Council of Advisors on Science and Technology regarding combating antibiotic resistance.

(ii) Within 180 days of the release of the Action Plan and each year thereafter, the Task Force shall provide the President with an update on Federal Government actions to combat antibiotic resistance consistent with this order, including progress made in implementing the Strategy and Action Plan, plans for addressing any barriers preventing full implementation of the Strategy and Action Plan, and recommendations for new or modified actions. Annual updates shall include specific goals, milestones, and metrics for all proposed actions and recommendations. The Task Force shall take Federal Government resources into consideration when developing these proposed actions and recommendations.

(iii) In performing its functions, the Task Force shall review relevant statutes, regulations, policies, and programs, and shall consult with relevant domestic and international organizations and experts, as necessary.

(iv) The Task Force shall conduct an assessment of progress made towards achieving the milestones and goals outlined in the Strategy in conjunction with the Advisory Council established pursuant to section 4 of this order.

Sec. 4. Presidential Advisory Council on Combating Antibiotic-Resistant Bacteria. (a) The Secretary of HHS (Secretary), in consultation with the Secretaries of Defense and Agriculture, shall establish the Presidential Advisory Council on Combating Antibiotic-Resistant Bacteria (Advisory Council). The Advisory Council shall be composed of not more than 30 members to be appointed or designated by the Secretary.

(b) The Secretary shall designate a chairperson from among the members of the Advisory Council.

(c) The Advisory Council shall provide advice, information, and recommendations to the Secretary regarding programs and policies intended to: preserve the effectiveness of antibiotics by optimizing their use; advance research to develop improved methods for combating antibiotic resistance and conducting antibiotic stewardship; strengthen surveillance of antibiotic-resistant bacterial infections; prevent the transmission of antibiotic-resistant bacterial infections; advance the development of rapid point-of-care and agricultural diagnostics; further research on new treatments for bacterial infections; develop alternatives to antibiotics for agricultural purposes; maximize the dissemination of up-to-date information on the appropriate and proper use of antibiotics to the general public and human and animal healthcare providers; and improve international coordination of efforts to combat antibiotic resistance. The Secretary shall provide the President with all written reports created by the Advisory Council.

(d) Task Force agencies shall, to the extent permitted by law, provide the Advisory Council with such information as it may require for purposes of carrying out its functions.

(e) To the extent permitted by law, and subject to the availability of appropriations, HHS shall provide the Advisory Council with such funds and support as may be necessary for the performance of its functions.

Sec. 5. Improved Antibiotic Stewardship. (a) By the end of calendar year 2016, HHS shall review existing regulations and propose new regulations or other actions, as appropriate, that require hospitals and other inpatient healthcare delivery facilities to implement robust antibiotic stewardship programs that adhere to best practices, such as those identified by the CDC. HHS shall also take steps to encourage other healthcare facilities, such as ambulatory surgery centers and dialysis facilities, to adopt antibiotic stewardship programs.

(b) Task Force agencies shall, as appropriate, define, promulgate, and implement stewardship programs in other healthcare settings, including office-based practices, outpatient settings, emergency departments, and institutional and long-term care facilities such as nursing homes, pharmacies, and correctional facilities.

(c) By the end of calendar year 2016, the Department of Defense (DoD) and the Department of Veterans Affairs (VA) shall review their existing regulations and, as appropriate, propose new regulations and other actions that require their hospitals and long-term care facilities to implement robust antibiotic stewardship programs that adhere to best practices, such as those defined by the CDC. DoD and the VA shall also take steps to encourage their other healthcare facilities, such as ambulatory surgery centers and outpatient clinics, to adopt antibiotic stewardship programs.

(d) Task Force agencies shall, as appropriate, monitor improvements in antibiotic use through the National Healthcare Safety Network and other systems.

(e) The Food and Drug Administration (FDA) in HHS, in coordination with the Department of Agriculture (USDA), shall continue taking steps to eliminate the use of medically important classes of antibiotics for growth promotion purposes in food-producing animals.

(f) USDA, the Environmental Protection Agency (EPA), and FDA shall strengthen coordination in common program areas, such as surveillance of antibiotic use and resistance patterns in food-producing animals, inter-species disease transmissibility, and research findings.

(g) DoD, HHS, and the VA shall review existing regulations and propose new regulations and other actions, as appropriate, to standardize the collection and sharing of antibiotic resistance data across all their healthcare settings.

Sec. 6. Strengthening National Surveillance Efforts for Resistant Bacteria. (a) The Task Force shall ensure that the Action Plan includes procedures for creating and integrating surveillance systems and laboratory networks to provide timely, high-quality data across healthcare and agricultural settings, including detailed genomic and other information, adequate to track resistant bacteria across diverse settings. The network-integrated surveillance systems and laboratory networks shall include common information requirements, repositories for bacteria isolates and other samples, a curated genomic database, rules for access to samples and scientific data, standards for electronic health record-based reporting, data transparency, budget coordination, and international coordination.

(b) Task Force agencies shall, as appropriate, link data from Federal Government sample isolate repositories for bacteria strains to an integrated surveillance system, and, where feasible, the repositories shall enhance their sample collections and further interoperable data systems with national surveillance efforts.

(c) USDA, EPA, and FDA shall work together with stakeholders to monitor and report on changes in antibiotic use in agriculture and their impact on the environment.

(d) Task Force agencies shall, as appropriate, monitor antibiotic resistance in healthcare settings through the National Healthcare Safety Network and related systems.

Sec. 7. Preventing and Responding to Infections and Outbreaks with Antibiotic-Resistant Organisms. (a) Task Force agencies shall, as appropriate, utilize the enhanced surveillance activities described in section 6 of this order to prevent antibiotic-resistant infections by: actively identifying and responding to antibiotic-resistant outbreaks; preventing outbreaks and transmission of antibiotic-resistant infections in healthcare, community, and agricultural settings through early detection and tracking of resistant organisms; and identifying and evaluating additional strategies in the healthcare and community settings for the effective prevention and control of antibiotic-resistant infections.

(b) Task Force agencies shall take steps to implement the measures and achieve the milestones outlined in the Strategy and Action Plan.

(c) DoD, HHS, and the VA shall review and, as appropriate, update their hospital and long-term care infectious disease protocols for identifying, isolating, and treating antibiotic-resistant bacterial infection cases.

Sec. 8. Promoting New and Next Generation Antibiotics and Diagnostics. (a) As part of the Action Plan, the Task Force shall describe steps that agencies can take to encourage the development of new and next-generation antibacterial drugs, diagnostics, vaccines, and novel therapeutics for both the public and agricultural sectors, including steps to develop infrastructure for clinical trials and options for attracting greater private investment in the development of new antibiotics and rapid point-of-care diagnostics. Task Force agency efforts shall focus on addressing areas of unmet medical need for individuals, including those antibiotic-resistant bacteria CDC has identified as public and agricultural health threats.

(b) Together with the countermeasures it develops for biodefense threats, the Biomedical Advanced Research Development.

Authority in HHS shall develop new and next-generation countermeasures that target antibiotic-resistant bacteria that present a serious or urgent threat to public health.

(c) The Public Health Emergency Medical Countermeasures Enterprise in HHS shall, as appropriate, coordinate with Task Force agencies' efforts to promote new and next-generation countermeasures to target antibiotic-resistant bacteria that present a serious or urgent threat to public health.

Sec. 9. International Cooperation. Within 30 days of the date of this order, the Secretaries of State, USDA, and HHS shall designate representatives to engage in international action to combat antibiotic-resistant bacteria, including the development of the World Health Organization (WHO) Global Action Plan for Antimicrobial Resistance with the WHO, Member States, and other relevant organizations. The Secretaries of State, USDA, and HHS shall conduct a review of international collaboration activities and partnerships, and identify and pursue opportunities for enhanced prevention, surveillance, research and development, and policy engagement. All Task Force agencies with research and development activities related to antibiotic resistance shall, as appropriate, expand existing bilateral and multilateral scientific cooperation and research pursuant to the Action Plan.

Sec. 10. General Provisions. (a) This order shall be implemented consistent with applicable law and subject to the availability of appropriations.

(b) Nothing in this order shall be construed to impair or otherwise affect:

(i) the authority granted by law to an executive department or agency, or the head thereof; or

(ii) the functions of the Director of the Office of Management and Budget relating to budgetary, administrative, or legislative proposals.

(c) This order is not intended to, and does not, create any right or benefit, substantive or procedural, enforceable at law or in equity by any party against the United States, its departments, agencies, or entities, its officers, employees, or agents, or any other person.

(d) Insofar as the Federal Advisory Committee Act, as amended (5 U.S.C. App.) (the "Act"), may apply to the Advisory Council, any functions of the President under the Act, except for that of reporting to the Congress, shall be performed by the Secretary in accordance with the guidelines issued by the Administrator of General Services.

BARACK OBAMA

THE WHITE HOUSE,
September 18, 2014.

INDEX

E

F

G

H

I

J

K

L

M

T

U

V

W

Y